Lacan on Depression and Melancholia

Lacan on Depression and Melancholia considers how clinical, cultural, and personal understandings of depression can be broken down and revisited to properly facilitate psychoanalytical clinical practice.

The contributors to this book highlight the role of neurotic conflicts underlying depressive affects, the distinction between neurotic and psychotic structure, the nature of melancholia, and the clinical value of Freudian and Lacanian concepts – such as object *a*, the Other, desire, the superego, sublimation – as demonstrated *via* a variety of clinical and historical cases. The book includes discussions of bereavement and mourning, transference in melancholia, suicidality and the death drive, excessive creativity, melancholic identification, neurotic inhibition, and manic-depressive psychosis.

Lacan on Depression and Melancholia will be essential reading for psychoanalysts and psychoanalytic psychotherapists in practice and training, Lacanian clinicians, and scholars of Lacanian theory.

Derek Hook is an Associate Professor of Psychology and a clinical supervisor at Duquesne University, Pittsburgh, USA, and a Extraordinary Professor of Psychology at the University of Pretoria, South Africa.

Stijn Vanheule is a clinical psychologist and a Professor of Psychoanalysis and Clinical Psychology at Ghent University, Belgium. He is also a privately practicing psychoanalyst and a member of the New Lacanian School for Psychoanalysis.

"In our contemporary world, depression is a substantial clinical problem. Yet, its conceptualization is vague, which is a crucial part of the problem. In this volume Hook and Vanheule collect papers that provide a refreshing Lacanian reading of depressive suffering, discussing how it takes shape in psychosis and neurosis, and how it reflects a specific position towards speaking, transference and the drive".

– **Paul Verhaeghe**, Psychoanalyst

"Written by trusted names in the field, this collection offers a uniquely Lacanian perspective on depression and melancholia, exploring the difference that a Lacanian approach offers both in understanding etiology and cure. The texts offer subtle clinical and theoretical explorations, offering something to the clinician and scholar, student and professional alike".

– **Kristen Hennessy**, Psychotherapist

This invaluable collection brings together the best of what can be said about depression from a Lacanian orientation. This is an indispensable collection for anyone interested in depression and its relation to the Freudian concept of melancholia, and one that should rightly be taken a launch pad for essential work to come.

– **Calum Neill**, Professor of Psychoanalysis & Cultural Theory

This collection links conceptual rigor in terms of Freudian-Lacanian psychoanalytic thought with contemporary clinical reality, addressing the failure of a culture that biologizes human suffering and is over-reliant on psychopharmacological and behavior-based methods of treatment. This book creates a social bond between clinicians, scholars, laypeople and those who engage in treatment, providing a cultural critique of the failure of identificatory bonds in a society hell bent on identity as a solution to existence. Melancholia is no longer restricted to "an illness" to cure, but a potential mode of subjective response recalling death to a ferocious social demand for limitless productivity and connectivity.

– **Manya Steinkoler and Vanessa Sinclair**, Psychoanalysts

Today's predominant socio-medical discourse aims to reduce intrapsychic conflict and suffering into an orderly diagnostic list of Disorders. Vague catch-all terms like depression lure in those craving the latest evidence-based quick-fix. This book, comprising papers by eminent Lacanian thinkers, promises no quick-fixes. Instead, it questions and critiques this discourse, reminding us that subjective complexity cannot be wished away by statistic conformity to some imaginary conflict-free Order. Highly recommended.

– **Christos Tombras**, Psychoanalyst

Lacan on Depression and Melancholia

Edited by Derek Hook
and Stijn Vanheule

Routledge
Taylor & Francis Group

LONDON AND NEW YORK

Designed cover image: Thierry De Cordier
MER HAUTE, 2011
oil paint on panel
170 × 105 cm
66 7/8 × 41 3/8 in

© Thierry De Cordier
Courtesy of the Artist and Xavier Hufkens, Brussels
Photo by: Dirk Pauwels

First published 2023
by Routledge
4 Park Square, Milton Park, Abingdon, Oxon OX14 4RN

and by Routledge
605 Third Avenue, New York, NY 10158

Routledge is an imprint of the Taylor & Francis Group, an informa business

British Library Cataloguing-in-Publication Data
A catalogue record for this book is available from the British Library

ISBN: 9781032106526 (hbk)
ISBN: 9781032106533 (pbk)
ISBN: 9781003216391 (ebk)

DOI: 10.4324/9781003216391

Typeset in Times New Roman
by Deanta Global Publishing Services, Chennai, India

To Stephen Frosh and Paul Verhaeghe, two inspiring mentors and teachers of psychoanalysis whose guidance, leadership and ongoing encouragement played its part in making this project - and many others - possible.

Contents

Contributors

Leon S. Brenner is a research fellow at the International Psychoanalytic University (IPU) Berlin, Germany, and the Hans Kilian und Lotte Köhler Centrum (KKC) at Rühr University Bochum, Germany. His work draws from the Freudian and Lacanian traditions of psychoanalysis, and his interest lies in the understanding of the relationship between culture and psychopathology. He is the author of *The Autistic Subject: On the Threshold of Language* (2020) and practices psychoanalysis in Berlin, Germany.

Joachim Cauwe is a teaching assistant at the Department of Psychoanalysis and Clinical Consulting, part of the Faculty of Psychology and Educational Sciences, Ghent University, Belgium. He obtained a Ph.D. in Psychology and a Pg.Cert in Psychoanalytic Psychotherapy in Freudian-Lacanian perspective from Ghent University. He works as a psychoanalytic psychotherapist in private practice.

Patricia Gherovici is a psychoanalyst, supervisor, and recipient of the Sigourney Award. She is the author of more than 70 articles and book chapters. Her books include *The Puerto Rican Syndrome* (2003, Gradiva Award and Boyer Prize); *Transgender Psychoanalysis: A Lacanian Perspective on Sexual Difference* (2017), and, with Chris Christian, *Psychoanalysis in the Barrios: Race, Class, and the Unconscious* (2019, Gradiva Award and American Board and Academy of Psychoanalysis Book Prize).

Russell Grigg practices psychoanalysis in Melbourne, Australia. He is a member of the Lacan Circle of Australia, the New Lacanian School, the École de la Cause Freudienne, and the World Association of Psychoanalysis. He has translated several of Lacan's seminars into English.

Derek Hook is an Associate Professor and clinical supervisor in Psychology at Duquesne University, USA, and an Extraordinary Professor of Psychology at the University of Pretoria, South Africa. He is the author of *A Critical Psychology of* *the Colonial* (2011) and *Six Moments in Lacan* (2017). Along with Calum Neill, he co-edits the Palgrave Lacan Series. He is also the co-editor of *Lacan and Race* (with Sheldon George), and the co-editor (with Calum Neill and Stijn Vanheule) of the landmark *Reading Lacan's Écrits* series. He maintains a YouTube channel including many lectures on Lacanian psychoanalysis.

Darian Leader is a psychoanalyst working in London and a member of the Centre for Freudian Analysis and Research. His books include *What Is Madness?*, *Hands* and *Why Can't We Sleep?*

Geneviève Morel is a psychoanalyst in Paris and Lille. She's a member of CRIMIC (Paris-Sorbonne) and CFAR (London), President of Savoirs et clinique and Collège de Psychoanalystes – A.l.e.p.h. She directs a clinical seminar in l'UHSA (CHU-Lille). Her books include *Ambiguïtés sexuelles. Sexuation et psychose* (2000), published in English as *Sexual Ambiguities* (2011), *Clinique du suicide* (Érès, 2002/2010), *L'œuvre de Freud. L'invention de la psychanalyse* (2006), *La loi de la mère. Essai sur le sinthome sexuel* (2008), published in German as *Das gesetz der Mutter* (2017).

Thomas Svolos practices psychoanalysis in Omaha, Nebraska. He is a member of Lacanian Compass, the New Lacanian School, and the World Association of Psychoanalysis. Svolos currently serves as a Professor of Psychiatry and Associate Dean for Strategy and Accreditation at the Creighton University School of Medicine, USA. Svolos is the author of *The Aims of Analysis: Miami Seminar on the Late Lacan* (2020) and *Twenty-First Century Psychoanalysis* (2017). He is co-editor of *Lacan and Addiction: An Anthology* (2011). His writings have appeared in nine languages.

Stephanie Swales is an Associate Professor of Psychology at the University of Dallas, USA, a practicing psychoanalyst, a licensed clinical psychologist, and a clinical supervisor located in Dallas, Texas. She has authored two books: *Psychoanalysing Ambivalence with Freud and Lacan: On and Off the Couch* (2019), co-authored with Carol Owens, and *Perversion: A Lacanian Psychoanalytic Approach to the Subject* (2012).

Stijn Vanheule is a clinical psychologist and a Professor of Psychoanalysis and Clinical Psychology at Ghent University, Belgium. He is also a privately practicing psychoanalyst and a member of the New Lacanian School for Psychoanalysis. He is the author of *The Subject of Psychosis: A Lacanian Perspective* (2011) and *Psychiatric Diagnosis Revisited – From DSM to Clinical Case Formulation* (2017). Together with Derek Hook and Calum Neill he is co-editor of the landmark *Reading Lacan's Écrits* series.

Jamieson Webster is a psychoanalyst in New York City and Part-Time Faculty at the New School for Social Research, USA. She is a founder of the psychoanalytic collective *Das Unbehagen* and a member of the Institute for Psychoanalytic Training and Research. She is the author of *Conversion Disorder* (2018), *The Hamlet Doctrine* (2013) with Simon Critchley, and *The Life and Death of Psychoanalysis* (2011). With Marcus Coelen, she is currently writing, *Remains to Be Read: On Jacques Lacan.*

Introduction

The failings of depression – A Lacanian orientation

Derek Hook and Stijn Vanheule

According to the World Health Organization (WHO) (2021), the total number of people suffering from depression is approximately 280 million, that is, 3.8 percent of the global population (5.0% of adults and 5.7% of adults older than 60 years). Depression, according to WHO, is a leading cause of disability worldwide and is a major contributor to the overall global burden of disease. These are concerning facts, and we need to bear in mind that some population studies indicate that the WHO numbers are an underestimation. For example, in the United States, the 12-month prevalence is probably as high as 10.4% and the lifetime prevalence is 20.6% (Hasin *et al.*, 2018). It comes as no surprise then that, along with anxiety disorders, depression is the most frequently diagnosed of all mental health ailments, and that a staggering amount of popular literature – memoirs, biographies, self-help texts – has been devoted to this topic. Depression, whether approached as a diagnostic label, as the epicenter of a spiraling socio-medical/biopolitical discourse, a mode of experience, or as a familiar cultural narrative, is omnipresent. It has become, both clinically and sociologically, an unavoidable concept, or, as we might put it in Lacanian terms, a *master-signifier*: an amorphous and encompassing term, used by so many people, in so many different ways, that it has become virtually impossible to dislodge, to effectively question or critique.

And yet, questioning and critique are precisely what is most urgently required. Despite enormous investments in research and evidence-based treatments, the prevalence of depression has not diminished over time – over the last decades, its impact only increased (World Health Organization, 2017). This failure challenges the pertinence and relevance of the dominant frameworks within which depression is studied – particularly biological and cognitive psychological models – just as it accentuates the crisis of how contemporary society functions. Indeed, as has often been observed, and as the WHO (2021) affirms, vulnerable societal subgroups suffer more severely from depression than privileged ones.

What then do Lacanian psychoanalysts have to offer when it comes to the conceptualization and treatment of depression? At first glance, the answer appears to be: not much. Jacques Lacan only referred to depression passingly, in a few isolated comments. This is not particularly surprising, both because the term falls short of the clinical and conceptual rigor required of a properly Freudian concept,

DOI: 10.4324/9781003216391-1

and because, in Lacan's time, this diagnostic label had not attained the pervasive cultural predominance it has today. Even when we move from Lacan's texts to a consideration of the secondary literature, we find that the term is still not frequently used by Lacanians. Overview works like the 2012 *Scilicet* volume of the *École de la Cause Freudienne* (2012) discuss it briefly, but reference texts like the *Dictionary of Lacanian Psychoanalysis* (Evans, 1996) don't mention it at all. The term remains a conspicuous absence from the index of most introductory and commentary texts on Lacanian psychoanalysis. Depression, in short, does not feature as a central concept within Lacanian psychoanalysis.

There are, of course, some notable exceptions to this conspicuous omission of reference to depression in the work of several Lacanian analysts (e.g., Chemana, 2012; Crosali Corvi, 2010; Leader, 2008; Lolli, 2022; Miller, 2008; Soler, 2016; Svolos, 2017; Vanheule, 2004; Verhaeghe, 2004). While the literature of this sort has certainly proved eager to engage and explore clinical phenomena behind the label of depression, it typically adopts a critical stance on how this concept is generally deployed. The consistent critique offered in such texts is that depression is a too-vague and too-overused term to afford either diagnostic precision or much by the way of clinical utility. (One might consider, by way of comparison, the careful analysis Freud affords the notion of melancholia, which, by contrast, *can* be considered a properly Freudian concept.)

Depression, as it is used as a catch-all term in everyday speech, seems, more than anything else, to refer to the malaise and discontent that many suffer as a result of living within the cultural conditions of the early 21st century. To address this area of suffering and work with the myriad of related issues that such subjects are confronted with, Lacanian analysts and scholars have needed to deconstruct and dissect the concept of depression. This alerts us to one of our key agendas here, namely, that of breaking down the numerous associated problems that have been bundled into this label into relevant material for psychoanalytic clinical work. Part of this work involves revisiting and refining the notion of melancholia (a focus of many of the chapters that follow), particularly in relation to issues of mourning, bereavement, and, more unexpectedly perhaps, creativity. How though have clinicians and theorists in the Lacanian tradition gone about this work of deconstructing and re-elaborating themes about the discourse of depression? An overview of the various chapters in this book will help us answer this question. However, before moving onto this task, we should pause to ask: What, most fundamentally, motivates the distrust and critique of Lacanians in respect of contemporary notions of depression?

Depression as a reductive concept

One doesn't need to look far to find some strong Lacanian views on the notion of depression. Skriabine (1997) advances, for example, that "The [Lacanian] psychoanalytic clinic refutes any idea of an entity that could be named *depression*". Such a blunt assertion might sound like a radical – and not entirely helpful

– position especially given today's many calls to recognize the disabling and often under-reported effects of depressive suffering. Nevertheless, this seemingly antagonistic stance to the routine and unquestioned use of depression as an all too ready-to-hand descriptive label has much to teach us.

Of the various critical vantage points that a Lacanian position affords us when it comes to the notion of depression, let us begin with a critique of the overuse of medication. The ever-expanding use of pharmacological medication certainly has much to answer for in the massive increase in diagnoses of depression, and, by extension, in the overuse of the concept of depression. As Etchegoyen and Miller (1996) argue, the utilization of drugs to alleviate people's overall feelings, results in the erosion of clinical phenomena, which fade out – or in some insistences, simply *continue to persist* – without ever having been properly understood or, indeed, *analyzed*. The end result of this is, invariably, the conflation of different symptoms, most typically "under the name of *depression*" (1996, p. 24).

Lacanian criticisms of the notion of depression expand here into a broader type of social critique. Consider Fink's comments:

> [T]he fact that people are increasingly diagnosed as depressed may ... reflect the simple fact that pharmaceutical companies have concocted ever more antidepressants, and when you have a "cure" you have to find a "disease" that can be treated with it – this is a ... widely documented problem in modern American culture ... . If doctors are convinced by pharmaceutical company representatives that they can cure depression with a pill, then doctors will be more inclined to label patients as depressed than as ... conflicted with themselves about love and hate they feel for [their] parents, for example ... But drug companies have no pill for "intrapsychic conflict" so it isn't likely doctors would be tempted to list it as a diagnosis.
>
> (2014, p. 246)

Therefore, following this logic, depression, as a diagnostic label, is more a marketing tool than a precise or particularly useful concept for clinical work. Given the widespread medical and pharmacological use of the concept, it is unsurprising that people go on to experience various difficulties in their lives in terms of the discursive category of depression. However, the labeling of experience as depression might, itself, be a means of aggravating symptoms that may have otherwise been interpreted – and worked with – quite differently.

We should be careful here in qualifying Lacanian critiques of pharmacological intervention. It is certainly true that many Lacanians take a dim view of what they would consider to be the over-prescription of medications for depression. "I see plenty of patients who come to me after having been diagnosed with depression and placed on a half-dozen different medications", says Fink (2014, p. 246), adding that "They usually get off the majority of medications fairly quickly ... [when] it becomes clear that the depression is the effect of longstanding neurotic conflicts" (p. 246). So, while there may, of course, be times when pharmacology plays a necessary role in the life of an individual, we should note the crucial Lacanian point: the particularities of a person's personality and the unique historical conditions of their life are all too often lost when it comes to pharmacological interventions. It is for this reason that the refutation of the popular notion of depression – as a malady to be treated by medications – has become tantamount to an ethical issue for many Lacanians. Indeed, the contemporary extension of the term depression can thus be seen as a symptom of discontent *within contemporary Western culture*. Leader (2008) disputes the idea that depression should be seen as a unique disease, and argues that the term should be jettisoned as a technical or diagnostic term, used merely as a descriptive term to refer to *surface features* of a behavior. Part of what drives Leader's critique of contemporary notions of depression is his concern with a culture that medicalizes solutions to problems of human suffering. In contemporary treatments of depression, he contends,

> [t]he interior life of the sufferer is left unexamined ... Depression ... is conceived of as a biological problem like a bacterial infection, which requires a specific biological remedy. Sufferers have to be returned to their former productive and happy states ... the exploration of human interiority is being replaced with a fixed idea of mental hygiene.
>
> (2008, p. 2)

Leader's is a position that prioritizes subjective meaning and the role of intersubjective relations over the reduction of apparent instances of depression to a biological or neurological state. Leader's (2008) argument, however, goes one step further. The objectification of a biological/medicalizing approach can, in effect, be an exacerbating part of the problem itself. Or, to word things in slightly stronger terms, today's conceptualization of depression could itself be considered to be iatrogenic. How so? Here, it helps to cite Leader (2008) at length:

> As so many different aspects of the human condition are explained today in terms of biological deficits, people become emptied of the complexity of their unconscious mental life. Depression is deemed to be the result of a lack of serotonin rather than a response to experiences of loss and separation. Medication aims to restore the sufferer to the optimal levels of social adjustment and utility, with little regard for the long-term causes and possible effects of their psychological problems.
>
> (Leader, 2008, p. 2–3)

Viewing depression as a localized disturbance that can be removed through targeted interventions overlooks the fact that such forms of suffering involve the whole of a given person's existence. Depression is not, as such, extricable from the domain of human and unconscious meaning. Separating states of depression from the everyday realm of lived experience and objectifying it in terms of medical language (as a bio-medical condition) undercuts the subject's own attempts to make sense of it, or to investigate the multiple facets of their personal history that may underpin it.

Added to this line of critique is the 'quick-fix' problem so evident in today's popular culture. We return here to the ethical quandary noted above – the problem of losing sight of the texture of subjectivity – which becomes more pronounced the more individuals are subjected to socio-medical norms:

> the more that society sees human life in ... mechanistic terms, the more that depressive states are likely to ramify. To treat depression on the same model as, say, an infection requiring antibiotics, is ... dangerous. The medicine will not cure what has made the person depressed in the first place, and the more the symptoms are seen as signs of deviance or unadapted behavior, the more the sufferer will feel the weight of the norm, of what they are supposed to be.
>
> (Leader, 2008, p. 3)

The discourse of depression engenders societal norms that many individuals fail to live up to. Similarly, depression once approached along the lines of medical and neurochemical interventions, that is, without the accompanying exploration of the patient's internal life, leads to expectations of a direct solution. In both such instances, the concept of depression can be said to be iatrogenic, to increase the sufferings of those who are unable to meet such social norms or such expectations of recovery.

In terms of Lacan's discourse theory (more specifically, the discourses of the master, the university, the hysteric, the analyst, and of capitalism), this focus on depression bears witness to the dominance of capitalist discourse. The societal omnipresence of depression is a collective attempt to try to ignore the 'sexual non-rapport', that is, the dimension of the 'real', understood here as a constitutive discordance, as the inescapable lack of integration, harmonization, or wholeness underlying not only the human sexual function but inter-subjective relations and the social link as such. Depression, understood in this way, is likewise an attempt to bypass the dimension of the unconscious that affects each human being (Vanheule, 2016). Social forms of ignorance take shape by focusing on solutions that aim at covering over a malaise, calming a type of political disorder or distemper, a move which proves ultimately unwarranted since the distemper itself signals to the subject that there is a margin within which they are free to live.

The deterioration of speech

Having sketched in broad strokes many of the most salient Lacanian critiques of how the notion of depression reduces the complexity of human subjectivity, we turn now to focus on a series of clinical issues. This is imperative because it makes clear that Lacanian attacks on discourses of depression involve more than just a critique of medical consumption culture. There are at least two fundamental reasons why depression is not accorded the status of a concept in Lacanian theory.

Firstly, the notion of depression is considered to be under-defined and too all-encompassing. As Hill (2002, p. 43) stresses, "the 'depression' of ordinary language and psychiatry is too vague a term". We can extend this: not only is the notion of depression lacking in specificity and conceptual refinement, but it also obstructs the work of more careful clinical listening. Skriabine (1997) affirms this when he comments that the notion of depression "covers certain particular sufferings with … [a] non-differentiating cloak". Indeed, what is sometimes labeled depression is, in some patients, far more akin to a state of nervous agitation; indeed, to a pronounced condition of anxiety (Leader, 2008). In other cases, 'depression' serves as a kind of proxy term, a synonym for the sadness, disappointment, or apathy that overwhelms an individual or a family. Lacanian clinical work breaks with this vagueness and aims at addressing the concerns that provoke these affects directly. If affective experiences overwhelm the body, this indicates that speech has been particularly powerless in articulating the subject and/or in keeping *jouissance* at a safe distance. This twin imperative, of expressing the subject and mediating *jouissance*, is nicely described by Gueguen (2009):

> in the treatment of depression and the prevention of suicide, we admit the phenomena inventoried by the empiricist doctrine (sadness, self-devaluation, etc.) but we do not isolate them from the whole of the state of the patient. The speaking being who addresses us is a whole. He is first of all a being of language: if he suffers today from what the DSM calls depression, if he has suicidal thoughts, they result from a very special entanglement, which is old although it may have been recently reactivated, between language and the regulation of the *jouissance* of the body.
>
> (2009, p. 11)

Depression, understood in this way, indicates a particular difficulty – i.e., a failure to use language in addressing the Other. Under such circumstances, speech, in its 'babbling' role of verbalization, often continues to be active, but the position of the Other *qua* structuring symbolic force is no longer properly operative. Words no longer structure an individual's position in respect of time, space, social circumstances, and life events. This type of speech fails to moderate *jouissance*. 'From this viewpoint', continues Gueguen (2009, p. 11), 'depression and [the] suicidal passage to the act will be considered according to our paradigm as diseases of disconnection [*débranchement*] of the social bond'.

In clinical practice, such states of disconnection call out for reconnection – this is exactly the challenge the analyst and patient are confronted with:

> The mood, the thymic disorder, translates the fact that the subject of the unconscious no longer finds in language and in the social bond the means to regulate, to pair [*d'appareiller*] with his body's drive *jouissance*. The first gesture of care will therefore be to allow a transference to be established, that

is, a bond of speech and confidence between the caregiver and the person treated. We see how the use of speech is at the forefront.

(Gueguen, 2009, p.11)

Gueguen goes on to conclude:

the essential thing is to help the subject to get out of the entanglements and impasses from which his body suffers when his relationship with language and truth is too hampered. The objective is not so much an unveiling of truth in itself, but an invention in the relationship of the subject with language which restores the desire and the possibility of action and of the social bond.

(Guegen, 2009, p. 12)

This brings us to a second crucial reason why Lacanians avoid the use of depression as a diagnosis.

Why affect is not a viable diagnostic indicator

Intensities of affect – and of so-called 'negative affect' – take on a great many forms. They often present as of focal and immediate importance in clinical work. Despite this, such affective intensities are not, in and of themselves, an indication of diagnostic structure. They are not useful, diagnostically, since they do not help the clinician grasp how the suffering subject is structured through 1) their use of language, 2) their relation to the Other, and 3) their attempts to manage *jouissance*. Clinically, this quickly becomes apparent: it is difficult, under the umbrella of depression, to properly discriminate between different types of depressive experience. For such differentiations, we need, instead, to turn to the three clinical structures specified by Lacanian theory: neurosis, psychosis, and perversion. It is for this reason that Lander argues:

From the point of view of psychiatric nosology, depression is a definite clinical entity. It is conceptualized through a group of phenomenological data that constitute a diagnostic clinical entity. [Lacanian p]sychoanalytic clinical practice, on the other hand, sees depression in a different way – as a symptom that is instated in any clinical structure. Depression is not an unconscious structure in itself.

(2006, p. 120)

In short: depressive phenomena should be seen as symptoms that can occur in any structure. This seems evident if we note that, despite apparent surface similarities in affective complaints, neurotic depression is ultimately very different in its underlying structural features from melancholia (typically referred to as psychotic depression). The unconscious and the drive have very different statuses for the subject in each of these conditions.

Fink adds a crucial qualification here noting that, in the context of neurosis, depression is more often than not the effect of longstanding conflicts. Accordingly, it is the conflicts that should be focused on, "not the affect, which may even at times be a ... smokescreen ... behind which the conflicts disappear from sight. *Affect is an effect, not a cause*" (2014, p. 246). To avoid a possible misunderstanding: Fink is not suggesting that *what appears* as depression is not clinically serious. He suggests – and this is a hallmark of Lacanian approaches more generally – that clinical diagnosis and conceptualization should dig deeper than affect, and should explore structure rather than behavioral/affective symptoms.

Verhaeghe (2004) extends this point, noting also how, from a Lacanian perspective, issues of identification are typically more *structurally* important than are questions of surface affects:

> Contemporary popular approaches focus on the affect and people quickly come to associate depression with certain negative emotions. But this is not the crux of it, quite the opposite in fact ... feelings – are deceptive. At the heart of depression, as is clinically not hard to see, is a lack of emotion, and a confrontation with emptiness and the loss of meaning ... . Depression can thus be conceived as the reverse of identity acquisition, the loss of an identificatory anchoring point ... In this way, depression is an essential possibility for every subject.
>
> (2004, pp. 274–275)

Verhaeghe supplies an intriguing clinical formula (depression as the reverse of identity acquisition) even as he stresses that we are all potentially susceptible to depressive suffering. Here again, though, a diagnostic distinction must be noted. In psychosis too, such a loss might occur, but whereas in neurosis depression signals conflict and subjective division, in psychosis – and in melancholia – it is indicative of a massive invasion by senseless *jouissance* that cannot be managed with the resources of language. In psychosis, the unconscious is a force that is experienced from *without* as opposed to from within (as in the case of neurosis). As such, an intimate interpretative stance that neutralizes the drive – an analytical strategy ideally suited to the treatment of neurosis – will prove ineffective. The linguistic processes that neurotics have at their disposal *via* various aspects of repression (chiefly, the metaphoric operations of condensation, the metonymic operations of displacement, and various aligned defenses) are not available in the same capacity in psychosis. To tackle psychotic forms of depressive experience and to counteract the impact of foreclosure, additional measures that counterweight *jouissance* are needed.

These diagnostic themes and the distinction between neurosis and psychosis (indeed, between neurotic depressive experience and melancholia) will be revisited several times in the chapters that follow. Our contributors explain how neurotic repression and psychotic foreclosure shape depressive complaints; they discuss how, from a clinical point of view, psychoanalytic work can address unconscious and *jouissance*-related issues. As will become abundantly apparent: restoring a relationship with the Other is crucial in this process, a consideration that speaks to the ongoing role of the speaking cure. We will turn shortly to an overview of the book's various chapters. Before doing so, however, we need to address an apparently scandalous comment that Lacan makes on sadness and depression in his televised comments in 1974 (later published as *Television* (Lacan, 1990)):

> People qualify sadness as depression by basing it on the soul [...]. But it is not an emotion [*état d'âme*: literally, state of the soul], it is simply a moral failing [*faute*: crime, fault, misconduct, offense, wrongdoing], as Dante, and even Spinoza, put it: a sin, which implies moral cowardice, which in the final analysis can only be situated on the basis of thought – that is, on the basis of the duty to put it well or to find one's way about in the unconscious, in structure.
>
> (1990, p. 22).[1]

Several factors should be considered in weighing up this remark. First, there is Lacan's aim of provocation, his wish to not only challenge his audience but also to overturn an accepted point of wisdom (namely that depression should be considered a type of illness). Second, we need to bear in mind Lacan's preference here for historical theological, Christian, and literary texts (Aquinas, Plato, Spinoza, Dante, etc.) above those of the social scientists and psychiatrists of his own time. References to such ancient and religious writings have a distinctive import on Lacan's theorizations, as Soler (2016) notes. It enables a very different conceptualization of the human subject as opposed to what was enabled *via* reference to the popular philosophical texts of the time.

The description of depression as a moral failing has a clear precedent in religious thought; the idea of sadness as sin had been debated for centuries, particularly as of offense to faith and God's love (Soler, 2016). The crucial underlying idea is that sadness can be thought of as sin, once we have realized that we are called by God, firstly, and that hope and joy are duties that stem from this calling, secondly. As Soler (2016) explains:

> [Sin] is an offense to God's charity, as Aquinas, for example, says regarding "acedia" ... [this] idea that sadness ... is the most serious sin ... comes from the theological views of the Church fathers ... Nevertheless, it is from Spinoza that Lacan borrows the idea of a sin that can be situated only on the basis of a thought, more precisely the idea that thinking clearly resolves sadness. This thinking clearly, which is the ... type of knowledge for Spinoza whose affect is joy, implies a whole conception of the relationship to a god who is ... equated with the cosmic order – one might, by analogy, say with the structural order.
>
> (2016, p. 69)

Lacan's reference to religious and theological texts facilitates a shift from the register of psychiatric thought to the ethical domain, hence the reference to the subject's duty "to find one's way about in the unconscious, in structure" (2001, p. 526). This duty is proper to analytical discourse, for, as Soler insists, "duties, like ethics, always being relative to a discursive order" (2016, p. 69). This duty, moreover, involves treating affect *via* the signifier, that is – to draw on the terms of Spinoza's philosophy – by means of the attempt to 'think clearly' *via* an engagement with the universal (or structural) order.

Whether addressed by Aquinas, Dante, or Spinoza, the theological topic of sadness, says Soler (2016), always implies a sin against the Other. This Other may vary; for Spinoza the Other is akin to the universal order, whereas, for Aquinas and Dante, this Other more closely approximates the locus of speech. In either case, this relation of sadness or joy to the Other, even though it is broached in religious terms, is of paramount importance. Indeed, as Soler asks:

> How could psychoanalysis – which operates by transference, in other words, by the hypothesis of the subject-supposed-to-know, which is one of the names of the Freudian unconscious but also one of the names of … God – not be more essentially concerned with [such religious ideas]? … Since Freud's time, this god has been the analysand's partner, who is assumed to harbor the signifiers that the latter deciphers in his own speech with the analyst's help.
>
> (pp. 70–71)

We are now in a better position to understand how Lacan's use of this idea from Christian ethics (the idea of depression as a moral failing) is importantly reinflected. The duty of which Lacan speaks is neither a duty to God nor to the life of a Christian: it is a duty *to speaking*, to putting one's life and troubles into speech, a duty in relation to the unconscious. Or, to put things differently, depression *can* be "a moral failing" if we shirk the responsibility of responding ethically (that is, clinically, *via* procedures of speech and relation to the Other) to depressive suffering. It can be a "moral failing" if we refrain from the exploration of the unconscious conditions of subjectivity. Lacan's provocative equation (depression/sadness as moral failing) can thus be read as an insistence on the need to explore – *via* the modality of the speaking cure – the specificity of a given manifestation of depression, which is always particular to a given individual's history and embedded within the culture and society of which they are a part. As Franco Lolli puts it, in his remarks on Lacan's above-cited remarks, depression can be approached

> as an impasse of the subject when faced with the task of going to the bottom of his/her own issues. The subject closes [themselves off] … in a kind of … refusal to know … The responsibility of the subject, to whom Lacan in [a] clear countertendency to the 'welfare' approach of modern psychology, calls the reader, is that of knowledge, of *bien dire* [saying it well]; the subject has

the ethical duty to seek the reasons for his/her suffering, to discover his/her implication in the symptom of which he/she complains.

(2022, p. 185)

It seems clear from this whose 'moral failing' Lacan is predominantly concerned with, it is the sufferer of sadness/'depression' themselves upon which responsibility is conferred. This is an irreducible aspect of Lacan's comments, one which cannot be denied, certainly so given that a central facet of Lacan's clinical ethics (Lacan, 1992) is to *avoid* a renunciation of responsibility for one's own subjective position (Neill, 2014).

We might expand upon this locus of responsibility, however, and, by circling back to many of the critical comments noted above, suggest that the moral failing and responsibility in question concerns – at least in part – our own current medicalizing, quick-fix, cultural milieu which invariably reduces the complexity of the subject and marginalizes the role of speech, subjective history and the transferential relation (to the Other) in its treatment regimes. In other words, depression as a master-signifier and psychiatric concept, is *itself* a moral failing insofar as it typically precludes an adequately ethical response to treatment. A culture that invariably biologizes loss, conflict and bereavement fails us by not considering these sufferings within the broader ambit of the subjective, personal historical and unconscious factors which underlie its particular manifestations.

To put this in more concrete terms, we might ask: why, exactly, is a given person unhappy, or 'depressed'? Perhaps they lost a loved one before a long-standing conflict could be resolved; maybe they have been subject to a lifetime's worth of racist degradation; possibly they are dealing with chronic pain on a daily basis; perhaps they have experienced an inexplicable malaise of personal value and meaning despite that everything else in their life had seemed to be running smoothly. What is to be stressed then, from a Lacanian position, is that there is not one biological/neurological entity called depression, but multiple historical, subjective, and unconscious antecedents to the sufferings of loss, bereavement, and depressive suffering, all of which should be approached *via* attention to the mediums of human experience, subjective meaning, and inter-subjective speech.

We turn now to an overview of the book's contents.

Chapter 1: Stephanie Swales: "Depression Reconsidered: The Well-Spoken, Neurotic Conflicts, and Desire'": Swales helpfully extends several of the basic arguments introduced above. She notes that depression has long been considered one of the most frequently occurring psychopathological diagnoses, observing also that it is widely recognized as a clinical syndrome by clinicians, researchers, and the general public. From a Lacanian perspective, however, depressed affect and the complaints that correspond to it are descriptive of someone's suffering and cannot be said to have a "real" or material existence that causes and explains its own existence. Diagnosis, for Lacan, Swales reminds us, is not based on descriptions of this or that maladaptive pattern of feeling, thinking, and/or behaving, but instead is *structural* in nature. As such, depression is not a discrete diagnosis but rather a way of naming the surface features of suffering that could be experienced by someone with any of Lacan's three main diagnostic categories of neurosis, perversion, and psychosis. Swales offers several ways of understanding the phenomenon of depression in neurotic individuals from a Lacanian standpoint. She first explores Lacan's claim in *Television* (1974/1990) that depression is the result of a moral fault. Second, she discusses how depression often serves to cover up repressed conflict. Third, she shows how depression can be indicative of a subject having given up on her or his desires.

Chapter 2: Stijn Vanheule: "In between the Signifier and the Real: On Depressive Experiences". This chapter continues the discussion of depressive suffering as it occurs in the neurotic structure. Vanheule begins his chapter by invoking the difficulty/movement matrix presented by Lacan (2014) in the first session of Seminar X. He then introduces a series of phenomenological descriptions to show how neurotic depressive trouble can be conceptualized as a combination of inhibition, emotion, and dismay (that is, with reference to the three successive terms on the vector of movement, in Lacan's matrix). Thus, Vanheule shows how the subject remains, in varying ways, immobilized in the symbolic in relation to the movement evoked by the drive (the top-to-bottom vector of movement, as Vanheule notes, indicates a force of movement that immobilizes the subject). The subject's discontent thus remains fundamentally unsignified, at least in the sense of not being properly integrated into the signifiers of the Other (the left-to-right vector of difficulty denotes the strength of this integration). More precisely yet: inhibition can be linked to the general immobility of the depressed subject; emotion to the overwhelming affective experience of sadness and despair; and dismay to the feeling of being deficient and generally impotent at the level of action. Through illustrations from Lacan's clinical practice (as reported by Lacan's analysands), Vanheule shows how clinical work with depressive subjects can be conceptualized as consisting of deliberate attempts to install symbolization in relation to a symbolic Other and by means of the metaphorical naming of discontent.

Chapter 3: Russell Grigg: "Forgetting and Remembering". Grigg begins by foregrounding a dilemma related to mourning. Mourning challenges the bereaved with two contrary imperatives. The grieving subject needs to work through the loss of a libidinal attachment while also being required to reinstate the memory of the loved one. How then might the process of mourning attend to both of these apparently opposed imperatives of remembering and forgetting? The symbolic process that provides the best means of responding to both of these imperatives simultaneously is memorialization. How though do we properly memorialize? For Grigg, it is the combination of ritual as a community event with the individual's psychical work of mourning that proves crucial; in this way, an effective form of commemoration can be achieved. However, there is also a *real* dimension to mourning, and it is here that a crucial difference between mourning and melancholia should be pinpointed. The work of mourning involves the transformation of the various imaginary features of the loved one into signifiers to be lodged in the Other, the process, in Grigg's words, of "the fall of the semblants".

As the imaginary features of the loved object fall away, one is partially exposed to the traumatic – or *real* – aspect of object *a*, the object cause of one's desire. The pain of this process, considerable as it may be, can be attenuated in mourning. This is not the case in melancholia, where the melancholic subject finds themselves defenseless against the traumatic real dimension of object *a*. This is an object which cannot be mourned, which remains forever in place, in an unmediated form. The melancholic is thus left confronting the grimace of the object which persists, exposed, like the grimace of a skull behind a beautiful face.

Chapter 4: Darian Leader: "Some Thoughts on Mourning and Melancholia". Freud's (1917) "Mourning and Melancholia" contains several contradictions, unexplored questions, and avenues for further research. Leader's chapter guides us through various aspects of Freud's landmark paper, highlighting several of its most interesting inconsistencies and implications before turning to the most significant analytical responses to it, namely those of Abraham, Klein, and Lacan himself. Lacan's views on the mourning process, particularly as conceptualized with reference to Hamlet in his fifth seminar (*Desire and Its Interpretation),* provide a useful resource in this regard. Leader argues that Klein and Lacan both seem to have been converging on particular aspects of mourning that help us situate the clinical phenomena with greater clarity. Leader also revisits the difference between mourning and melancholia, noting that "Mourning ... involves the process of establishing the denial of a positive term" whereas melancholia, by contrast, "involves the affirmation of a negative term". The melancholic subject is, for Leader, in two places at once, split between the 'unreal' world of social being and their 'real' existence of absolute solitude. Given that these two spaces cannot be superimposed, the melancholic confronts an impasse of communication: how might this agony be communicated? Only, it would seem, *via* figurative types of reference. Hence, perhaps, the frequency of recourse to descriptions of heaven, hell, or purgatory in various historical eras. Such descriptions can have a formative impact on the experience of the melancholic, providing an expressive framework for melancholic despair.

Chapter 5: Stijn Vanheule: "Conceptualizing and Treating (Manic-Depressive) Psychosis: A Lacanian Perspective". Starting from the hypothesis that psychosis makes up a structure with a precise status for the unconscious, Vanheule's second chapter explores how, from a Lacanian point of view, the treatment of psychosis is organized. As Vanheule argues, special attention needs to be paid to the specificity of the psychotic symptom and the way transference characteristically takes shape in such cases. The occurrence of psychotic symptoms bears witness to a subjective crisis, in which no signifiers provide support. This is particularly so when the subject is forced to deal with fundamental self-directed epistemic questions ("Who am I?") and questions concerning the intentionality of the other ("What do you want?"), as they rebound at the level of the unconscious. Characteristically, such questions are organized around intimate topics like dealing with parenthood and authority; life in the light of death; sexuality in relation to love and procreation; and sexual identity. Psychotic crises are triggered upon confrontations with such issues in daily life, where no support by means of a master-signifier or Name-of-the-Father can be found. It is crucial, from a Lacanian standpoint, that the psychoanalyst aims at restoring a place for the subject in relation to the Other, something which is typically threatened in episodes of acute psychosis. Vanheule draws on clinical material from Lacanian work with a female patient suffering from manic-depressive psychosis, to illustrate these ideas.

Chapter 6: Joachim Cauwe and Stijn Vanheule: "Maneuvers of Transference in Psychosis: A Case Study of Melancholia". This chapter extends the discussion of psychotic structure, arguing that psychosis is characterized by non-separation from the object *a*. As the authors explain, transference in psychosis consequently remains at the level of duality and appears to take on an inverted form, where it is *the Other* that looks for something in the patient and not *vice versa*. This, understandably, makes the handling of transference challenging since there is no evident triangular structure that can mediate between the patient and the Other. Moreover, the patient cannot rely on the Other to deal with difficult experiences of *jouissance* marked by excess and senselessness. Cauwe and Vanheule ground the above conceptualizations by referring to the details of clinical work with a patient suffering from melancholic psychosis. They highlight three important forms of intervention in the case, each of which provided a space where the clinician could maneuver within the transference in order both to avoid the development of persecutory or erotomaniac relations and to provide the possibility of finding solutions in dealing with psychic suffering. The first of these interventions involved locating the clinician as a non-threatening 'little' other (as opposed to the position of a big symbolic Other). The second focused on interpreting the 'mad' Other. The third involved developing an interest in the patient's affinities and favored activities.

Chapter 7: Derek Hook: "The Complex of Melancholia". Hook's chapter explores key facets of melancholia by referring both to a clinical case and *Into the Wild*, Jon Krakauer's memorable (1996) book (the inspiration for Sean Penn's well-known film of the same name) depicting the tragic story of Christopher McCandless. Hook foregrounds a series of clinical themes that may be grouped under the general theme of problems in symbolic fixity: difficulties in receiving gifts; the inability to mediate relations of intimacy; yearning for anonymity/ disappearance; and experiences of the twilight world. These themes, while perhaps not obviously associated with Freud's account of melancholia, nonetheless represent areas of diagnostic priority for a Lacanian approach attuned to the role of symbolic processes and the intrusive traumatic *real* object. Hook also highlights the role of the death drive in melancholia. He stresses that a different set of conceptual priorities comes to the fore in a Lacanian as opposed to a Freudian conceptualization of the death drive, particularly considering Lacan's insistence on the death drive as involving both facets of symbolic mortification and "undead" life (or *jouissance*). Such an approach to the death drive, which entails both the desire to break from the symbolic roles, debts, and obligations that structure social existence, and the drive to attain a type of life in excess of life, proves illuminating when applied to the clinical case and to the Christopher McCandless story.

Chapter 8: Geneviève Morel: "Susan Stern: Sham". "[S]tudying a single case can … be instructive or even paradigmatic, as it gives us a glimpse of something more universal". This is how Morel opens her chapter with an account of the melancholic revolutionary figure, Susan Stern. Stern was a member of the militant Leftist US 1960s organization, the Weathermen, who, during the Vietnam War, called for armed struggle against the American State. In the view of Susan's ex-husband, Robby Stern, the Weathermen provided a social and political pretext for Susan's pre-existing suicidal tendencies. Many of the details of her autobiography – carefully analyzed by Morel – confirm this suggestion. Multiple facets of her life resonate with clinical cases of melancholia. Stern speaks, for example, of quasi-hallucinatory visions, epiphanies of death. Her descriptions of her body as a corpse suggest an identification or – as Morel puts it – a "communion" with the dead, which, paradoxically enough, brings her, for a short time, out of depression. As Morel remarks, Stern's self-appointed and derisory nickname, Sham, materialized her super-egoic contempt for herself, as did her descriptions of herself as a "worm, disgusting, foul". More telling yet were Stern's multiple suicide attempts – the first at 13 years of age – her self-proclaimed obsessions with death, dying, murder and violence, and her wish to be killed, preferably in a blaze of revolutionary glory. Stern's apparent goal – "*To sacrifice everything*: her possessions, her ego, her image, her female identity and finally even her name" – amounted to a radical expression of the death drive, which for Freud, as we know, exists in a near pure state in melancholia. What Stern was looking for in extremist ideology, argues Morel, was a solution to a severe and possibly psychotic existential divide, an ideal image, an identity that could unite her violent and sexual drives with her political ideals. For a short time, Stern managed to reconcile this painful split; the ideal image of the female revolutionary magnetized Stern, provided her with "divine inspiration". Ultimately, however, this unifying image proved unsustainable, especially so in the context of the onslaught of a punitive superego that pushed her toward suicide.

Chapter 9: Leon S. Brenner: "Excessive Creativity in Melancholia". Brenner's chapter introduces a series of Lacanian contributions to thinking about melancholia, mourning, and creativity. A crucial part of Brenner's discussion includes invoking and explaining several fundamental Freudian and Lacanian concepts, such as: the object cause of desire (*objet petit a*); the ideal ego and ego-ideal; sublimation; the lack in the Other; and das Ding. Melancholia is described as an excessive creative process, which exhausts the subject's capacity to desire and which results in their breaking libidinal ties with the world. Given that melancholia occurs within a psychotic structure, it necessarily entails a form of foreclosure. However, as observed by Brenner, the foreclosure at work in melancholia is of a particular sort: it involves both radical reference to an object that is originally and constitutively lacking and also identification with this loss. This impossible endeavor brings about the debasement of the ego as well as something akin to suicide on the part of the object. Following Giorgio Agamben, Brenner proposes that melancholia should not be viewed as a pathological form of mourning but rather as a unique creative process that aims to transform an unobtainable unknown object into a lost object. Through a consideration of Freud's and Lacan's theories of creativity, Brenner goes on to offer a metapsychological framework that explicates a type of excessive melancholic sublimation. Crucial here is the idea of a type of "negative" sublimation in which the ego runs the risk of becoming the object of the death drive. In this process, the subject betrays its reliance on the symbolic order and directs its creativity toward an impossible ideal, based on an overvaluation of the lost object. Accordingly, the psychoanalytic treatment of melancholia can be said to concern the construction of an imaginary "limit" to the hold of the impossible idealized object. More particularly yet, clinical work with melancholic subjects can be conceived as revolving around the mobilization of the dynamic qualities of the ideal ego in the imaginary, which function as a limit to the hold of the object cause of desire on the ego-ideal.

Chapter 10: Jamieson Webster and Patricia Gherovici: "Dressing up the Death Drive: Mourning as a Defense against Melancholia". Webster and Gherovici's chapter continues the exploration of the relationship between creativity, mourning, and melancholia. At first glance, creativity appears to be a form of mourning, whereas melancholia, by contrast, seems to necessarily entail the failure of sublimation. This distinction can be further developed: in mourning, we find an attempt at interiorizing the object, whereas in melancholia we find the *refusal* of mourning, the feeling of *being* the object and *not having* or interiorizing the object. Of course, what numerous examples—including the poetry of Sylvia Plath and the "ravaging beauty" of Alexander McQueen's fashion—quickly make obvious, is that a state of melancholia by no means precludes artistic production or creation. As such, and as Webster and Gherovici intimate, we need a more complex conceptualization of the distinction between mourning and melancholia in respect of creativity and artistic production. The status of the object is again crucial here. For the mourner, the *lack* of the object causes suffering; for the melancholic, as the authors put it, "the object of grievance is not ... lost but rather maintained within the subject, buried alive in the ego ... becoming a devouring vortex of pain". Without the loss of an object (object *a*), the operations of desire grind to a halt; it is for this reason that we see in melancholia, not just a refusal of mourning but of desire itself. "Self-laceration, the abnegation of the melancholic, is one attempt to introduce a cut, to encounter the scene of one's desire". Subsequently, in clinical work, the analyst might assist the melancholic analysand "by creating a hole, an interval, a space, to break ... the death drive's grip and allow the object *a* to be extracted". If this happens, there will be room for intervention, indeed, for a type of stable creation that does not merely fuel the self-destructive energies of melancholia. Lacan's notion of the *sinthome* proves useful here. As Webster and Gherovici point out: "The work of analysis implies not only a yielding of *jouissance*; it is not simply about the fall of an illusion or traversal of a fundamental fantasy but rather the constitution of something new, a *sinthome*, that is, the creation of a new symptom that does not need to be cured".

Chapter 11: Darian Leader: "The Specificity of Manic-Depressive Psychosis". Historically, Lacan only very rarely made reference to manic-depressive psychosis. This is perhaps unsurprising given that Lacanian theorizations of psychosis typically focus only on three variants of psychosis: paranoia, schizophrenia, and melancholia. Nevertheless, manic-depressive psychosis has been the focus of a great deal of psychiatric literature in the past, just as the current diagnostic category of bipolar has generated a spiraling body of literature in the present. Leader's chapter asks to what extent manic-depressive psychosis can be considered a viable diagnostic category from a Lacanian clinical standpoint. How, he asks, should manic-depressive psychosis be properly differentiated from mania and depression? Furthermore, in what ways does manic-depressive psychosis structurally resemble other variations of psychotic structure? By drawing on memoirs of manic-depression and utilizing case vignettes alongside salient examples from the history of psychiatry, Leader offers answers to these questions and identifies what is most distinctive about manic-depressive psychosis.

Chapter 12: Thomas Svolos: "Depression Screening as the Latest Avatar of Moralism in American Public Health". Svolos observes that depression screening has become standard practice in mental health environments, primary care clinics, schools, and workplaces across the United States. This has occurred, he notes, despite that there is little evidence supporting the value of the practice in terms of the recognition or management of depression. Svolos explores this topic from a number of critical perspectives. He questions not only the aligned roles of the Medical-Industrial Complex and large pharmaceutical companies but also the broader psycho-economic discourse of worker productivity which has seen, as he puts it, "an extension of the Taylorist doctrine into the minds of workers". As part of a succinct historical overview of various antecedents of depression screening, Svolos singles out Mental Health America, an organization that, despite its mission of promoting mental health, remains essentially a mental hygiene movement. The Lacanian dimension to Svolos' critique becomes apparent when he reminds us that moral reform efforts within the field of mental health – from the temperance movement and movements against sexuality to mental hygiene and depression screening – occur as part of the transition to monopoly capitalism. More than just this, such reform efforts involve an implicit appeal to an Aristotelian Sovereign Good, which is precisely what Lacan (1992) takes issue with in his *The Ethics of Psychoanalysis*, where he warns that analysts attempting to "establish the universal spread of [moral and consumer] goods … implies an amputation, sacrifices, indeed a kind of puritanism in the relationship to desire" (p. 303).

Acknowledgments

Thanks to Dany Nobus, the editor and founder of the *Journal for Lacanian Studies* (JLS), for graciously allowing us permission to reproduce two articles that were first published there (Darian Leader's "Some Thoughts on Mourning and Melancholia" and Stijn Vanheule's "In between the Signifier and the Real: On Depressive Experiences"). The contribution by Thomas Svolos "Depression Screening as the Latest Avatar of Moralism in American Public Mental Health' was first published in *Re-Turn: A Journal of Lacanian Studies* (2010) and is reprinted with permission. Thanks, in this respect, go to Ellie Ragland. We are indebted to the prior editorial work of Vanessa Sinclair and Manya Steinkoler who edited the book *On Psychoanalysis and Violence* (Routledge, 2018), which included Geneviève Morel's chapter "Susan Stern: Sham". We likewise acknowledge the editorial work of Patricia Gherovici and Manya Steinkoler on *Lacan on Madness* (Routledge, 2015), where Darian Leader's chapter, "The Specificity of Manic-Depressive Psychosis" was first published. Russell Grigg's chapter ("Remembering and Forgetting") first appeared in the online journal *LCExpress* (3, 2, 2015) many thanks to our two colleagues Azeen Khan and Thomas Svolos for granting us permission to reproduce that paper here. Joachim Cauwe and Stijn Vanheule's chapter "Maneuvers of Transference in Psychosis" originally appeared in 2018, as "Maneuvers of Transference in Psychosis: A Case Study of Melancholia from a Lacanian Perspective" in the *British Journal of Psychotherapy* (34, 3, 376–392). Many thanks to the publishers of this journal for permission to reproduce that article here. Stijn Vanheule's chapter "Conceptualizing and Treating (Manic Depressive) Psychosis", originally appeared in 2017 in the *British Journal of Psychotherapy* (33, 3, 388–398) under the title "Conceptualizing and Treating Psychosis: A Lacanian Perspective". Once again, thanks go to the publishers of this journal for permission to reproduce that article here. A special note of thanks also to John Dall'Aglio who offered both administrative and research assistance in the preparation of this manuscript.

Note

1   This specific translation of Lacan's (1990, p. 22) comments, with the additional translator's notes, is Bruce Fink's, and is included in Soler's (2016) text *Lacanian Affects* (2016, p. 99).

References

Chemama, R. (2012) *La Depression, La Grande Nérvose Contemporaine*. Toulouse: Erès.

Crosali Corvi, C. (2010) *La Dépression: Affect Central de la Modernité*. Rennes: Presses Universitaires de Rennes.

École de la Cause Freudienne (2012) *Scilicet: L'ordre Symbolique au XXIe Siècle*. Paris: ECF/Huysmans.

Etchegoyen, R.H. & Miller, J-A. (1996) *Silence Brisé*. Paris: Agalma.

Evans, D. (1996) *An Introductory Dictionary of Lacanian Psychoanalysis*. London & New York: Routledge.

Fink, B. (2014) *Against Understanding Volume 2: Cases and Commentary in a Lacanian Key*. London & New York: Routledge.

Freud, S. (1917). Mourning and Melancholia. In J. Strachey (Ed.), *The Standard Edition of the Complete Psychological Works of Sigmund Freud*, Volume XIV. London: Hogarth Press, pp. 237–258.

Gueguen, P-G. (2009) 'The Plunge of the Symptom in Hypermodernity', *Lacanian Compass*, 1, pp. 5–12.

Hasin, D.S., Sarvet, A.L., Meyers, J.L. et al. (2018) 'Epidemiology of Adult DSM-5 Major Depressive Disorder and Its specifiers in the United States', *JAMA Psychiatry*, 75, pp. 336–346.

Hill, P. (2002) *Using Lacanian Clinical Technique*. London: Press for the Habilitation of Psychoanalysis.

Lacan, J. (1990). *Television*. New York & London: Norton. (Original work published 1974)

Lacan, J. (1992) *The Seminar. Book VII: The Ethics of Psychoanalysis (1959–1960)*, trans. F. Last, ed. J.-A. Miller. London: W.W. Norton.

Lacan, J. (2001) *Television*. London: Norton.

Lacan, J. (2014) *The Seminar. Book X: Anxiety (1962–1963)*, trans. F. Last, ed. J.-A. Miller. Cambridge: Polity.

Lacan, J. (2017) *The Seminar. Book V: Formations of the Unconscious (1957–1958)*, trans. F. Last, ed. J.-A. Miller. Cambridge: Polity.

Lander, R. (2006) *Subjective Experience and the Logic of the Other*. New York: Other Press.

Leader, D. (2008) *The New Black*. London: Penguin.

Leader, D. (2015) 'The Specificity of Manic-Depressive Psychosis', In P. Gherovici & M. Steinkoler (Eds.), *Lacan & Madness: Yes, We Can't*. London & New York: Routledge, pp. 127–138.

Lolli, F. (2022) 'Depressions', In D. Busiol (Ed.), *Lacanian Psychoanalysis in Practice*. London & New York: Routledge, pp. 177–206.

Miller, J-A. (2008) 'Massive Propaganda to Track Down Depression', *Lacanian Ink*, 31, pp. 8–15.

Neill, C. (2014). *Without Ground: Lacanian Ethics and the Assumption of Subjectivity*. London: Palgrave.

Skriabine, P. (1997) 'Some Moral Failings Called Depression', *The Symptom*. Lacan.com. http://www.lacan.com/depression.htm

Soler, C. (2016) *Lacanian Affects: The Function of Affect in Lacan's Work*. London & New York: Routledge.

Svolos, T. (2017) *21st Century Psychoanalysis*. London: Karnac.

Vanheule, S. (2004) 'Neurotic Depressive Trouble: Between the Signifier and the Real', *Journal of Lacanian Studies*, 2, 1, pp. 34–53.

Vanheule, S. (2016) 'Capitalist Discourse, Subjectivity and Lacanian Psychoanalysis', *Frontiers in Psychology*, 7, 1948. https://doi.org/10.3389/fpsyg.2016.01948

Verhaeghe, P. (2004) *On Being Normal and Other Disorders: A Manual for Clinical Psychodiagnostics*. New York: Other Press.

World Health Organization (2017) *Depression and Other Common Mental Disorders: Global Health Estimates*. Geneva: World Health Organization. Licence: CC BY-NC-SA 3.0 IGO

World Health Organization. (2021) *Depression*. World Health Organization. Retrieved January 20, 2022, from https://www.who.int/news-room/fact-sheets/detail/depression

Chapter 1

Depression reconsidered

The well-spoken, neurotic conflicts, and desire

Stephanie Swales

Depression has long been considered one of the most frequently occurring psychopathological diagnoses, and it is widely recognized as a clinical syndrome (encompassing certain characteristic symptoms) by clinicians, researchers, and the general public. (In fact, in the DSM-5, depression is not one disorder but rather a cluster of related disorders, the depressive disorders, which are all supposedly different syndromes based on differences such as meeting a specified minimum number of symptoms in a category and the duration and severity of the suffering (APA, 2013).) However, as one of the main types of so-called "mood disorders", it may instead be seen as a diagnosis based on a reification of a flat or sad affect. From a psychoanalytic perspective, a depressed affect and complaints which correspond with it (e.g., difficulty sleeping or excessive self-recrimination) merely describe someone's suffering and cannot be said to have a "real" or material existence that somehow causes and explains its own existence (Vanheule, 2017). Neither is altered brain chemistry, such as a decrease in serotonin and norepinephrine, a cause, but instead is yet another form of description.

Diagnosis, for Lacan, is not based on descriptions of this or that maladaptive pattern of feeling, thinking and/or behaving, but instead is structural in nature. As such, depression is not a discrete diagnosis but rather a way of naming the surface features of suffering (Leader, 2008) that could be experienced by someone with any of Lacan's three main diagnostic categories of neurosis, perversion, and psychosis. These structures are based on certain characteristic ways of situating oneself in relation to the lack in the Other (for further explication see, for example, Fink, 1997). This article will consider several ways of understanding the phenomenon of depression in neurotic individuals from a Lacanian perspective. First to be explored is Lacan's claim in *Television* (1974/1990) that depression is the result of a moral fault. Second, is how depression often serves to cover over a conflict that has been repressed. Third, depression can be indicative of someone having given up on her or his desire. Clinical vignettes will assist in demonstrating these arguments.

Depression as a moral failing: as seen on television

Like any form of suffering available to lived experience, a depressed mood— whether sadness or "flatness"—can, especially in our society, be taken as the

DOI: 10.4324/9781003216391-2

manifestation of a glitch in one's neurological system. As such, depression is a meaningless annoyance that warrants pharmacological or psychological treatment that targets the surface symptoms and attempts to eradicate them as soon as possible. In Seminar XI (Lacan, 1964/1998), Lacan speaks of the initial status of the analysand in treatment characterized by a will-not-to-know or a passion for ignorance. From this position, the analysand asks the analyst to fix the problem, eradicate the suffering and return her or him to a former state of enjoyment, but without the patient having to do the work of exploring the unconscious. A New Yorker cartoon humorously depicts the everyday reality of a passion for ignorance: a wife and husband are sitting on opposite ends of a couch and the wife has presumably just asked her husband to tell her what he is thinking. He responds, "How should I know what I'm thinking? I'm not a mind reader" (Sipress, 2020). In the cartoon scenario, the complexity of neither conscious nor unconscious mental life is given its due. The analysis can only be said to have properly begun when this passion for ignorance is at least partially overcome by a superseding desire to know about the workings of one's unconscious. For instance, the analysand might begin to see dreams as meaningful or wonder why, despite being well-prepared for giving presentations at work, s/he always manages to forget some crucial piece of information.

In *Television*, Lacan said that depression is a "moral failing" or a "moral weakness, which is, ultimately, located only to thought; that is, in the duty to be Well-spoken, to find one's way in dealing with the unconscious" (1974/1990, p. 22). As such, the ethical duty of the Well-spoken is to overcome the passion for ignorance and to engage in the talking cure. To do so requires not just to speak but to be well-spoken; that is, to explore manifestations of the unconscious and to radically put oneself and one's symptoms into question. It follows that, in some cases, depression dissipates once the analysand is able to take up the ethical call to articulate her- or himself about life issues and manifestations of the unconscious. In these instances, insofar as the analysand continues beyond the falling away of the depression—often for years—with her or his treatment, we can see clearly that depression is not the sum of the problems from which the analysand suffers. The analysand at this point formulates more specific complaints about life and her- or himself which drive the analytic work forward.

For example, a middle-aged man sought treatment for what he had self-diagnosed as ADHD and depression. He listed the symptoms he was experiencing that corresponded with the symptoms he had read about online, including depressed mood, difficulty making decisions and concentrating, and feeling excessively guilty. He had never been to see a therapist before and imagined that he might learn some skills from me that would help him feel as happy as he felt was befitting of a man in his life situation. After all, he had a good job, a family, and a hobby, so what more could he ask for? Perhaps, he thought, I might refer him to a psychiatrist, and he could receive medication. After just a handful of sessions, to his surprise, what he had experienced as his depression and ADHD all but disappeared. Instead, he realized that he was experiencing significant ambivalence in several key areas of his life. To mention just one: although he knew his elderly father was increasingly unwell, he had been avoiding visiting him or even speaking to him on the phone, despite his best-laid plans to do so. He began to realize that he had used his depressed mood and accompanying bodily lethargy as an excuse not to visit his father and that his self-recriminations for being a bad son were, in part, tied to hateful thoughts about his father—thoughts which he knew he would have to face if he were to be face to face with his father. Avoiding contact with his father was also an indirect way of expressing his hatred. In sum, the clearing up of this man's depression went hand in hand with his seeing meaning in his depression and recognizing an unconscious conflict that he would spend the next stage of treatment resolving. He had shifted from a passion not to know, from wanting to be patched up and sent back to his life as it was, to following the ethics of the Well-spoken.

Depression as hiding a neurotic conflict

Emotions can be deceptive. In Freud's article "The Unconscious" (1915/1957), he said that when an idea is repressed and causes symptomatic effects, the affect associated with the ideational representative either continues to exist in its current form—although often it is displaced—or it is transformed into another affect. In other words, the formation of a neurotic conflict can result in a depressed mood. The depressed mood is therefore not the correct area of focus for clinical attention; uncovering the conflict that it conceals is where attention should be turned.

As Carol Owens and I have argued in our recent book, *Psychoanalysing Ambivalence with Freud and Lacan: On and off the Couch* (Routledge, 2019), ambivalence, about loved ones, for instance, is often poorly tolerated in our culture. In such conflicts, our hateful thoughts about a loved one are repressed, and the affect associated with it—hatred—is frequently transformed into a depressed affect (although it can also transform into anxiety or another affect). Depression, with its frequent companion of superegoic self-recriminations or "low self-esteem", can thus sometimes be seen as hatred for another turned around on the self. Indeed, in *Civilization and Its Discontents* (Freud, 1930/1961), Freud underlined that when aggressive thoughts are repressed, the superego responds by turning them against the individual in the form of guilt (p. 139).

A depressed, obsessional, neurotic patient with a characteristic complaint that it was "too late" (Lacan, 1958–1959/2019) for him to train for and obtain a successful job and start a family was in a relationship with an older woman past childbearing age and had been underemployed during the early months of the analysis. After much self-doubt and procrastination, he finally applied for and was offered a job that more fully utilized his qualifications. He found, to his surprise, that he was capable of performing the tasks he was assigned. However, he quickly felt dependent on the praise of his boss in order to motivate himself to do his work and, for the most part, procrastinated until the last minute by taking naps at work and otherwise doing nothing. Even when at home, he had trouble thinking of anything he wanted to do, so unless his girlfriend was around, he tended to nap or aimlessly surf the internet. He had frequent thoughts of being worthless and felt undeserving of the love of his girlfriend and the positive regard of his boss. The analysand was perplexed about all of this and could not understand his persistent depression because ostensibly things were better than ever for him with his job and his relationship.

He described his mother as "borderline" intrusive and controlling, and, for these reasons, he had cut off contact with her. As a child, however, he had experienced great pleasure at being picked out as her favorite from amongst his siblings. For many years, he had not made major decisions on his own and had tried to meet her every demand. She insisted he attend an elite private school for both grade school and college, and he felt great pressure to succeed academically. He later became aware of her controlling behaviors and resented her for it, often choosing the opposite of what she wanted from or for him. At the time of the analysis, he was initially convinced that he unambivalently hated his mother and wanted nothing to do with her, yet he chose not to block her number on his phone and would read the text messages she sent him. Much to his embarrassment, he spoke about sexual dreams that featured his mother. Thinking back on his interactions with her, he realized that his mother had sexualized their relationship, as, for example, she had been jealous of his girlfriends, and she spoke openly about her own body to him in a sexualized fashion. The analysand described one disturbing dream as follows:

I forced my mom onto her knees, grabbed her by her head and her hair. I put her cock in my mouth and forced her to get me off. It was all very satisfying to put her in her place.

The interpretation of the dream revealed the analysand's desire to force his mother onto her knees, a position of supplication, which was a reversal of what had been their power dynamic. He said he was unsure whether he wanted to make her beg for him to stop or to beg for more, and here he grappled with his sexual attraction to his mother and how his object choice (of an older girlfriend) in hindsight rendered this attraction apparent. Finally, his slip of the tongue—saying "I put her cock in my mouth" rather than "I put my cock in her mouth"—belied an ambivalence about which of them should have the phallus, who was the desiring subject, as well as which of them should be in the position of enjoyment and if he wanted to be the cause of her enjoyment or not.

Similarly, in terms of the Other's desire and *jouissance*, the analysand became jealous and resentful of his boss, who often took a vacation or worked from home. In response, to assert the freedom of his desire and his right to *jouissance* which he felt was threatened by that of his boss, the analysand frequently took sick days when he knew his boss was taking a vacation. The analysand's sleeping on the job or not working while at work was a way to avoid being in the position of sexual object for his mother and to avoid fulfilling her desires for him to work hard and succeed. In addition, although he derived some enjoyment from secretly slacking off and rebelling against the Other's desire, at the same time his superego had its say about this, thus keeping him depressed, feeling worthless, and unable to fully enjoy himself. His depressed mood may have resulted from transformed hatred as well as transformed love, as thoughts related to both affects were repressed. The analysand's depressed affect and corresponding self-castigation was a kind of compromise formation, such that it was both a disguised return of the repressed and operating via the superego to punish him for his repressed desires. Although, initially, he understood his depression as resulting from his inadequacies and chemical imbalances that manifested in low energy and anhedonia, through the process of analysis he discovered that it actually functioned to hide this spider's web of conflicts surrounding his mother.

In contrast, the depression of a hysterical analysand centered around her desire for unfulfilled desires and her avoidance of pleasurable *jouissance*. She was middle-aged, married with two children, and had a demanding career. She was unhappy in her marriage and, despite the fact that for many years they had not had sex, let alone shared romantic words, she said nothing to her husband about her complaints and desire for divorce, feeling very worried about hurting him and also worried that he would flare up in anger (even though he was a calm, generally approachable person). The analysand enjoyed romance novels and comedic films, but hid these preferences from others, rarely allowing herself to indulge in them, and instead trying to make herself read nonfiction books, watch documentary films, go to art galleries, and the like—all things she felt she should enjoy but did not enjoy. If she were at a friend's house and was asked if she would like something to drink, she found herself automatically saying she wanted nothing, even though this was false. She felt compelled to work harder and longer hours than anyone else in her company's department, despite recognizing that it was unnecessary and that she could succeed in her job without doing so. On one occasion, she received a text from her brother that featured her brother smiling and enjoying a relaxing vacation. The analysand said she felt a bit hurt that her brother was shoving his vacation in her face and that he did not ask how she was doing. She felt proud of herself for pushing her resentment aside and responding enthusiastically that she was glad her brother was enjoying his vacation. The analysand said she felt more depressed than usual in the days after this exchange and found herself ruminating on a chain of instances in which her family did not take what she wanted into account. At the same time, she recognized that she was perfectly capable of taking a vacation and that she was responsible for her relative lack of enjoyment. Even when she did take vacations, she recognized that she would often try to hide it from her friends and family, lest they accuse her of enjoying herself too much. She had this concern even though she structured her vacations so that she was often on work calls while her children and husband had fun.

The analysand felt guilty for having felt resentful at her brother and, in general, her depressed affect and self-deprecation served to cover over her anger and complaints about others. Her extreme fear of her husband's anger, for instance, was a projection of her own anger. Through the course of her analytic work, she began to realize how often she was angry at others, and that avoiding its direct expression was not sufficient to eradicate it; instead, it manifested in her depressed mood, self-hatred, and passive-aggressive actions toward the objects of her anger, such as not returning a phone call. Her efforts at resolving her underlying conflicts succeeded in eradicating her depression.

Depression as giving up on one's desire

In Lacan's seventh seminar on ethics, he commented that the only thing the subject can be guilty of is having given up on its desire (1959–1960/1992, p. 319). In this vein, we can understand, for instance, the aforementioned hysteric's guilt for not going on a vacation and not pursuing her desire with her marriage. The guilt that typically corresponds with subjective complaints of depression, then, may, in many cases of neurosis, indicate not following one's desire. Further, a depressed mood is often the affect associated with conflicts marked by giving up on one's desire.

In another case of hysteria, a woman became increasingly depressed living in a city she disliked, working as an executive in a company she helped to found and being married to a man who made her dread coming home from the work she disliked. In terms of her marriage, she complained that her husband was controlling and flew into interminable rages at the slightest of provocations. With each of these situations, she felt it was due to a moral failure on her part that she was having difficulty enjoying, or at least appreciating her situation. Why she wondered, could she not find something to love about her new city? Why could she not be proud of her business accomplishments and enjoy her new executive role instead of wishing she were in her former role in which she dealt more directly with clients? Why was she unable to communicate her desires to her husband in a way that could be more effective? Likewise, the analysand severely chastised herself for having gained weight. She imagined that if only she could eat more healthily and get back into a rhythm of regular exercise, she would feel more confident and as a result obtain the ability to take on the unsatisfying aspects of her life and turn them into positives. In a move typical of individuals in neoliberal society today, she reasoned that her unhappiness in work and love was due to her own insufficiencies. Correspondingly, she criminalized her desire and tried to conform to the Other's desire, attempting to obey various superegoic commands. At the inception of this woman's analysis, then, she demonstrated a passion for ignorance about her unconscious as well as having relinquished her desire, and her depression did not abate until she began to follow her desire.

To consider a case of an obsessional neurotic, a white man sought treatment after his long-term girlfriend broke off their relationship upon discovering his infidelity. He had a longstanding pattern of cheating on his partners, and he wanted to find a way to end the cycle. He suffered from terrible guilt and self-loathing and had been depressed for many months. At first, he felt he needed to learn better relapse prevention skills to control his behavior, but he soon became curious in his own unconscious and wondered about the meanings and function of his symptom of infidelity.

He had a history of getting and trying to get into relationships with women with whom he had been infatuated and who fit the perfect picture of an attractive white woman who might be featured, he said, in a Playboy magazine. Sometimes, he would chase after such a woman for years without his hopes coming to fruition. When he did enter into a relationship with a woman he pursued, he would inexplicably have trouble maintaining an erection during sexual acts but had no such troubles when masturbating with the aid of pornography.

During the last months of his relationship with his most recent ex, he had cheated on her with a black woman whom he found very attractive and with whom he had no trouble performing sexually. After the girlfriend ended their relationship, he did not feel much sadness or regret because he did not believe that he truly wanted to be in that relationship. This fact was of interest since he had initially said he fell into a depression as a result of his breakup. Instead, his depression materialized months later when he tried to start a relationship with the woman with whom he had been having an affair. The two of them got along very well and he admired her as a person in addition to having chemistry with her in the bedroom. He had organized a weekend getaway for the two of them, with the explicit intention of starting their committed relationship. However, when on the trip he found himself tortured by guilt and anxiety, and the two of them parted permanently. From that moment on, he felt deeply depressed and presumed his guilt was about having ruined his relationship with his ex, whom he then tried fruitlessly to convince to take him back. He decided there was something wrong with him that had damaged his relationship with the perfect woman that he should have married.

Through the process of analysis, the analysand came to realize that his "type" had always been black women and that, if he was honest with himself, he was not attracted to white women. Having grown up in a predominantly white, racist environment with racist parents, his desire for black women was formed in relation to the Other's desire. He had always felt deeply ashamed about his attraction to black women and tried his best to hide it not only from others but also from himself by pretending that his type was a white Playboy model look-alike. His attraction for black women was a way to rebel against, express aggression toward, and question the values of his parents, but he had not been able to openly avow these thoughts and desires. Later in the analytic work, he was disturbed by the racism inherent in this conflict.

The analysand realized that he had contrived their first date as a weekend getaway so that they would not be seen—as an interracial couple—by anyone in his social circle. Notably, the moment when he felt the object of his desire was attainable instead of impossible, that he could have a fulfilling relationship with her, was the moment he fled in anxiety, once again rendering their relationship impossible. His guilt, then, was not truly guilt for what he had done to his ex, nor was his depression due to having ruined his relationship with his ex. Instead, his depression and guilt were due to not following through with his desire and entering a relationship with the other, black woman.

Conclusion

As these clinical examples should make clear, the three underlying causes discussed for the surface symptoms of depressed mood and self-castigation are by no means mutually exclusive. Far from it, they often co-occur. In the case of the most recently discussed male analysand, his will-not-to-know anything about his unconscious had kept him in a cycle of repetition instead of remembering, and his avoidance of following the path of his desire was clearly related to repressed desires, to conflicts with his parents and with the Other. The resolution of his depression did not arrive until he made progress in all three realms.

As a final note, contemporary culture lends itself to the abdication of desire—and thus to the development of depression—via the capitalist discourse and the push for *jouissance* over desire. In the capitalist discourse, subjective lack is denied and the subject is lured to purchase yet another product, another S1, to supposedly fully remedy its discontents. For instance, when a parent's child moves out of the house to attend college, rather than mourning the loss, the parent purchases a new car. When mourning is ignored and covered over by reaching for an S1—be it a new car, a pint of ice cream, a new wardrobe, or anti-depressant pills (without also engaging in talk therapy)—it renders the subject susceptible to depression. Under the capitalist discourse, to attempt to solve the discontents of everyday life, the subject might seek job promotions, more money, or more luxurious vacations; each one ultimately fails to make the subject feel whole and perpetuates a tendency for depression insofar as *jouissance* is pursued at the expense of desire. Related is the idea that nothing is so successful in preventing pleasurable enjoyment and ensuring painful *jouissance* as the superegoic command of our day of "Enjoy yourself!" Contemporary depression, then, is often related to the denial of loss and of lack and the consequent abdication of the path of desire that is produced and reproduced in the discourse of the capitalist.

References

American Psychiatric Association. (2013) *Diagnostic and Statistical Manual of Mental Disorders* (5th ed.). https://doi.org/10.1176/appi.books.9780890425596

Fink, B. (1997) *A Clinical Introduction to Lacanian Psychoanalysis: Theory and Practice.* Cambridge, MA: Harvard University Press.

Freud, S. (1957) 'The Unconscious', In J. Strachey (Ed.), *The Standard Edition of the Complete Psychological Works of Sigmund Freud*, Volume 14. London: The Hogarth Press and the Institute of Psycho-Analysis, pp. 159–215.

Freud, S. (1961) 'Civilization and Its Discontents', In J. Strachey (Ed.), *The Standard Edition of the Complete Psychological Works of Sigmund Freud,* Volume 21. London: The Hogarth Press and the Institute of Psycho-Analysis, pp. 57–146.

Lacan, J. (1990) *Television (1974)*, trans. D. Hollier, R. Krauss, and A. Michelson. New York: W. W. Norton & Company.

Lacan, J. (1992) *The Seminar. Book VII: The Ethics of Psychoanalysis (1959–1960)*, trans. D. Porter, ed. J.-A. Miller. New York: W. W. Norton & Company.

Lacan, J. (1998) *The Seminar. Book XI: The Four Fundamental Concepts of Psychoanalysis (1964)*, trans. A. Sheridan, ed. J.-A. Miller. New York: W. W. Norton & Company.

Lacan, J. (2019) *The Seminar. Book VI: Desire and Its Interpretation (1958–1959)*, trans. B. Fink, ed. J.-A. Miller. New York: W. W. Norton & Company.

Leader, D. (2008) *The New Black: Mourning, Melancholia and Depression*. London: Penguin.

Sipress, D. (2020, April 27) [Cartoon]. Retrieved June 28, 2020, from https://www.newyorker.com/cartoons/issue-cartoons/cartoons-from-the-april-27-2020-issue

Swales, S. & Owens, C. (2019) *Psychoanalysing Ambivalence with Freud and Lacan: On and off the Couch*. New York: Routledge.

Vanheule, S. (2017) *Psychiatric Diagnosis Revisited: From DSM to Clinical Case Formulation*. London: Palgrave Macmillan.

Chapter 2

In between the signifier and the Real

On depressive experiences

Stijn Vanheule

Introduction

Epidemiological psychiatric researchers conclude that the lifetime prevalence rate
for major depression in the general population is between 12% and 17% (Angst,
1997; Lepine *et al.*, 1997). Although it is not clear whether depressive experiences are really more prevalent today than in previous times, it is indisputable that
subjective awareness of such experiences has increased (cf. Ehrenberg, 1998).
'Depression' is a popular signifier that circulates in our contemporary discourse.
It often functions as a '*point de capiton*' that organizes people's complaints.
It is a master signifier that speaks to people (Miller, 1996–97, session 21 May
1997). Consequently, psychoanalysts need to conceptualize the issue of depressive complaints, determine how they are constituted, and explore how they can be
approached clinically.

Lacan paid scant attention to the issue of depression and depressive complaints,
but this didn't prevent him (and many analysts following Lacan) from critically
appraising this umbrella concept. His most explicit commentary on depression
can be found in his 1974 booklet *Television,* (cf. Lacan, 1974/1990, p. 26) where
he criticizes the idea that it constitutes an illness. Through a reification of sadness
and by attributing to it the status of a condition, we mobilize the belief that it is
a disease or a disorder. Such interpretations are deceptive and misguided. They
engender the idea that depression is a hidden condition that needs to be treated
as such. Rather, like any affective state, depressive experiences should be studied
in terms of the encounter, or clash, between the body and speech. Speech affects
the body, and *vice versa*. Here, variation of its impact can be discerned, depressive experiences being just one of them. In *Television,* Lacan (1974/1990) suggests that depressive experiences coincide with a withdrawal from "the duty of
the Well-Spoken" (p. 26). Neglecting manifestations of the unconscious in one's
own functioning and refraining from articulating oneself as a subject in relation to
issues occurring in life, make up the breeding ground for depressive experiences.

This chapter will not go into a critique of the depression concept and its various failings but focus instead on the structure of *depressive experiences in neurosis*. To do so, we study Lacan's principal comment on depressive experiences

DOI: 10.4324/9781003216391-3

in *Television* in terms of the complex ground he sets ten years earlier (i.e., the difficulty/movement matrix) in Seminar X (Lacan, 1962–63) around the Freudian inhibition-symptom-anxiety tripartite (cf. Freud, 1926). In my reading, the left-hand column of the difficulty/movement matrix helps us to situate the position implied by depressive experiences, beyond the semiological characteristics observed by descriptive psychiatry. With the typical twist Lacan gives to the concepts under discussion, the matrix enables us to link depressive experiences more specifically to his basic idea that these problems are expressions of poor symbolic articulation. Moreover, I argue that this matrix enables us to clarify the clinical preliminary work that needs to be done in psychoanalytic sessions.

Phenomenological observations

Let us first go briefly into phenomenological observations of depression and melancholia made by Ey and Minkowski, Lacan's contemporaries and acquaintances in French psychiatry (Allen, 2001).

In their famous textbook on psychiatry, Ey *et al.* (1967) discern three core characteristics that constitute depression: sadness ('thymia', 'tristesse'), inhibition, and moral pain ('douleur morale'). Sadness, considered to be the most significant characteristic, is indicated by feelings of irritation, disgust, and despair. Inhibition implies a blockage or slowing down of mental and physical activities, resulting in withdrawal from others, fatigue, and an inability to act. Moral pain refers to self-accusation, self-punishment, pessimism, and feelings of guilt.

In the phenomenological approach, these experiential characteristics are typically connected to a general organizing principle, a specific being-there in the world (cf. Widlöcher, 1995, pp. 60–74; Fuchs, 2001) that, according to both Minkowski (1933) and Ey (1954), is based upon temporal disorganization. For them, depression is a malady of time and is linked to a suspension in the normal perception of time. This is manifested by a suspension of the distinction between past, present, and future and by the patient's impression that the course of time is inverted. Depression, accordingly, is conceived of as a situation of deceleration, stagnation, and monotony. Rhythm is lost, actions become paralyzed and inertia is the result.[1]

Although Lacan only touched upon these phenomenological observations,[2] in my interpretation, the left column of his difficulty/movement matrix contains an alternative framework for situating these components of depressive complaints.

The matrix

The difficulty/movement matrix is a simple, two-dimensional table with three columns and three rows, and arrows indicating the degree to which one is in the realm of the dimension concerned (see Figure 2.1). The table itself contains nine clinical manifestations, which attract attention because of their phenomenological[3] roots.

Difficulté / Difficulty: degree of structuring by the signifier

Mouvement /

Movement:

Drive intensity

Inhibition (Hemmung)	Empêchement Impediment	Embarras Embarrassment
Emotion	Symptôme Symptom	Passage à l'acte
Émoi Dismay	Acting-out	Angoisse Anxiety (Angst)

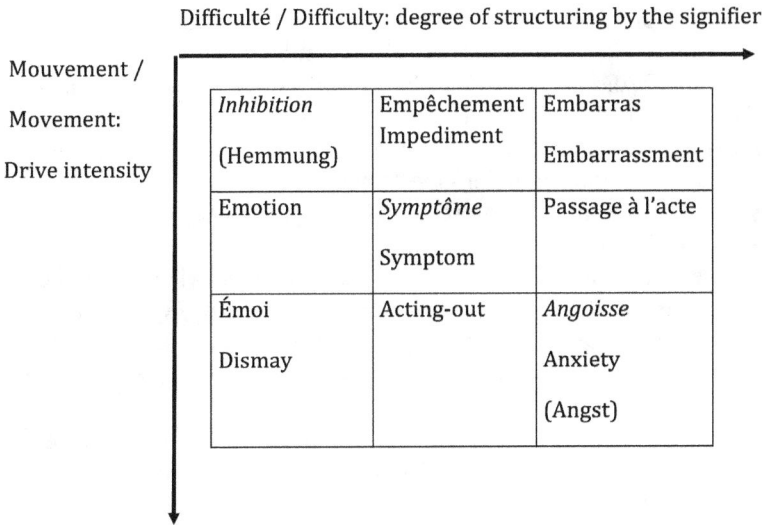

Figure 2.1 The difficulty/movement matrix

Crucial for our understanding of the Lacanian difficulty/movement matrix is the meaning of both vectors.[4]

Lacan (1962–63, p. 7) relates the idea of *movement* to Little Hans' phobic object: the horse that terrifies Hans by the racket it makes ('*Krawall machen*'). Movement is linked to the horse's rearing up, and to Hans' observation that horses fall down (cf. Lacan, 1994, p. 348). In line with this metaphor, the dimension of movement signifies the Freudian '*Triebregung*'; the pulsation of the drive that, at moments, floods the body. If we consider movement from the perspective of the four terms Freud (1915) associates with the drive – namely pressure, source, object, and aim – we can conclude that it concerns pressure ('*Drang*'), which Freud defines as a form of activity and as a 'motor moment'. Pressure signifies the degree of power and force implied by the tension of the drive. In Lacan's diagram, movement refers to drive intensity.

Using his own concepts, Lacan in the 1960s, suggests that, at the level of movement, the Real is pressing. For him, the quality of movement is essential to the Real (Lacan, 1964–65, 5 May 1965), and it presses when corporeal *jouissance* insists on our experience of the body.

In Seminar XX, Lacan returns to the question of movement, indicating that in Freud's oeuvre, the concept of movement is linked to excitation. It produces a *jouissance* that mobilizes the body in provocative ways: "excitation provokes movement with the aim of getting rid of it" (Lacan, 1975, p. 58, my translation).[5] If this fails, it implies a pressure that becomes increasingly unbearable.

The typical means through which we as humans respond to this surplus is the signifier and the Other; that is, the dimension of the symbolic and the various resources of speech and linguistic expression that come with it, but the solution that the signifier provides is only partial. The dimension of *difficulty* indicates this attempt to signify the intensity of the drive with which one is confronted at the level of the Real. It denotes the degree to which the movement of the body is articulated in terms of the signifiers of the Other. When speech is assumed in its structuring and castrating function, the Other is the place where we constitute ourselves as divided subjects. As soon as this happens, the dimension of the unconscious is constituted.

The right side of the difficulty vector indicates a situation where the Other is far too present ("too much of the signifier" [Lacan, 1962–63, p. 78]). In that case, there is a lack of lack – that is, anxiety – in the relation between the moved body and the Other, and suffering will take shape in relation to the Other's insisting desire.

The left side of the vector, on the other hand, implies a situation of 'not enough' ("too little of the signifier" [Lacan, 1962–63, p. 78]), where there is only minimal structuring by the signifier.

Drawing upon this difficulty/movement or signifier/drive matrix, one could say that a subject is a result of articulating the moved body in the intersection of the Real of the drive and the Other. Therefore, this positioning between both vectors also implies taking up a position in relation to the object *a* and, consequently, a particular constitution as a desiring subject. As early as the 1960s, Lacan considered the object *a* as the residue of corporeal *jouissance* that is divided by the Other, hence of castration. The object *a* is what remains left at the level of the body when the Real (cf. 'movement') meets with the Other (cf. difficulty), a leftover for which no signifier can be supplied: "as soon as something comes to knowledge, something is lost and the surest way of approaching this lost something is to conceive of it as a bodily fragment" (Lacan, 1962–63, p. 134). Indeed, a radical incapacity is inherent to all uses of the signifier, which Lacan highlights by attributing the quality of difficulty to the dimension of the Other.

In his discussion of the categories of the matrix, Lacan is mainly interested in the peculiarities of the subject's position towards the object *a*. This interest in the subject/object *a* relation distinguishes Lacan's approach from both a phenomenological one that sticks to the level of the 'Erlebnis' (experience) (Lacan, 1962–63, p. 163), and a general psychological or psychiatric approach that adheres to the reification of psychical experience. For Lacan, the logical relation between the subject and object *a* is anterior to all phenomenology.

Depression of the Other

We will now go into the three categories of the left column: 'inhibition', 'emotion', and 'dismay'. As indicated, I suggest that these categories reflect the structural position implied in depressive experiences. These categories are, respectively, the Lacanian counterparts of the phenomenological categories: 'inhibition', 'sadness', and 'moral pain'.

The three categories all reflect a relative absence of the Other, that is, increasing difficulty in the expressive use of the signifier at the vector of difficulty. Therefore, it could be argued that, in this case, *the symbolic Other is depressed* and, consequently, the *realization of the subject by way of a manifestation in chains of signifiers is in question.* Following this line of thinking, depressive trouble reflects an absence of the division and conflict that are inherent to the use of the signifier. The Real presses the affected body on the scene, but the latter hardly gets transposed in terms of articulated signifiers, which, in their turn, are produced as one aims to express what provoked the movement in the first place. The difficult work of articulating questions and ideas around the events and contexts that effect the subject has seized up. It is barely proceeding at all. The necessary movement is hardly even being brought into existence by the signifying chain, which is why the depressed person can barely manifest as the subject of the signifier. In Freudian terms, we could say, the afflicted subject lacks the necessary symbolic resources with which to begin the process of working through the affects they are suffering. This results in a stagnant position at the level of the Other. The circulation of signifiers and the signifying capacity of the Other are suspended. Therefore, language loses its metaphoric value in organizing reality. This can be clinically observed in the monotonous and empty discourse that is characteristic of depressive complaints.

A major consequence is that the depressive complaint points to a disturbing Real that is only loosely integrated into the Other. Thus, the characteristic depressive complaint of feeling like the outcast of a senseless world is quite accurate. The experience of being affected is signified poorly, and suffering is largely felt as a provocation at the level of the body.

When Lacan (1974/1990) designates depression as "a moral failing, ... which means a moral weakness ... in relation to thought" (p. 26), he remains within this line of reasoning. Here, again, the depressive complaint is considered to be remiss at the level of the signifier. The subject has defaulted in not making adequate use of speech as the unique means by which one manifests oneself as a subject.[6]

Inhibition, emotion, and dismay

The categories of inhibition, emotion, and dismay differ to the extent that they imply a different level of movement and a different position towards the object *a*. The categories imply a specific stance towards the most extreme category in the matrix, anxiety, and can be considered as a differing means of defending oneself against being overwhelmed by it.

The concept of *inhibition* was central to the theories of Herbart and Griesinger (cf. Smith, 1992). They were undoubtedly the source of the concept as Freud, their pupil, went on to apply it throughout his oeuvre (cf. Vanheule, 2001). Freud elaborates upon the concept most fully in 'Inhibitions, Symptoms, and Anxiety' (Freud, 1926), where he indicates the concept's relevance for developing an understanding of depressive states (*'Depressionszustände'*). He defines an inhibition as "the expression of a *restriction of an ego-function*" (Freud, 1926, p. 89) or as "a restriction of the ego's functioning" (Freud, 1933, p. 83) in defending against the pulsating drive ('*Triebregung*'). The ego-functions that can particularly become inhibited are the sexual function, eating, locomotion, and the ability to work (Freud, 1926). Lacan follows Freud by situating inhibition at the level of functioning but specifies the concept by linking it to the body ("Inhibition ... Is always a matter of the body" [Lacan, 1974–75, 10 December 1974, my translation]).

An inhibition indicates that someone *was* about to be overwhelmed by an unbearable impulse and fled from it. Lacan states that inhibition concerns a function that is contaminated by a displaced desire. Ego-related functioning might imply the choice to radically avoid this second desire and defend oneself against it by paralyzing the entire function. Inhibition is thus a mode of structural miscognition, a choice "not to see" (Lacan, 1962–63, p. 332). It blocks the possibility of being moved and of any symbolic articulation ("It makes up a bar ... against all that is articulated like the Symbolic" [Lacan, 1974–75, 13 May 1975, my translation]).

Since certain functions can be considered to be the domain wherein the drive's pressure manifests as circling the object *a* (cf. Lacan, 1973), inhibition threatens to break off the dynamic relation between subject and object, which normally guarantees a differentiation between both subject and object. One serious consequence that can arise from the effacement of this distinction is that desire is structurally blocked. A second consequence is that the articulation of the subject is suspended, which produces an experience of aimlessness. No longer structured by the Other, nor affected by the flux of movement, the subject risks being reduced to the nothingness and the numbness of an object *a* that is no longer encircled by means of the signifier. In such a case, one will at least partially identify with the position of the outcast ('déchet') (Lacan, 1975). Lacan (1962–63, p. 332) indicates that, clinically, this position of exclusion is risky since it can result in a *passage à l'acte*, such as suicide, whereby the subject effectively identifies with the nothingness of the object *a*.

The concept of *emotion* is interpreted quite literally by Lacan as an ex-motion: disintegration or disorder at the level of movement. As such, he distances himself from the psychological meaning that is attributed to emotion. For Lacan, emotion is the result of being confronted with a situation or a task one doesn't know how to deal with (Lacan 1962–63, p. 332: "misrecognition"). At the experiential level, this confrontation provokes a catastrophic experience: one does not know what to do; there is no signifier in the Other that could guarantee or orient, and thus support, the subject. Quite the contrary, since as 'emotion' corresponds to the confrontation with the radical lack in the Other, it implies a confrontation with the *obscurities* of the Other's desire. No common factor articulates the subject in relation to the enigmatic desire of the Other. Knowledge that enunciates a position towards the object *a* in relation to the Other is missing, which results in despair.

Lacan considers this situation, whereby an enigmatic surplus arises at the level of the Other's desire, to be a precipitating factor for a *passage à l'acte*. Because of the inability to use language (and linguistic operations such as metaphor and metonymy) as an anchoring point, there is always a danger that the imaginary stagnation turns into an unbearable situation, into a Real overturning.

In discussing the concept of *dismay* ('*émoi*'), Lacan first criticizes the French translation of '*Triebregung*' as '*emoi pulsionnel*' and indicates that a correct understanding of the concept requires studying its etymological roots. He traces the term back to the ancient French verbs '*émoyer*' or '*esmayer*' and to the Latin '*exmagare*', which all refer to 'to trouble oneself', 'to frighten', and 'to lose potency'.

Dismay is a matter of positioning oneself as being unable to act or respond, as being impotent. In dismay, one is, on the one hand, in a situation of being intensely moved, of experiencing a radical confrontation at the level of the Real. This situation calls for signifying articulation such that a desiring subject can manifest. On the other hand, full speech fails, which undermines the subject. Here, then, the object *a* violently erupts. To illustrate this situation, Lacan (1962–63, p. 312) refers to Freud's Wolfman, who freezes as he sees the wolves sitting in the tree in his dream. This dream in fact refers back to a similar reaction of paralysis as he witnessed the primitive scene between his parents. While this scene moved him intensely, he couldn't comprehend it (he lacked a signifier for it) and was thus unable to manifest himself as a desiring subject. In Wolfman's case, the accompanying emergence of the object *a* took place at the anal level – which is typically the case in obsessive neurosis.[7] Dismay can be observed in the little boy's defecation while witnessing the intercourse between his parents and in the later anal fixations of his desire.

In depression, dismay is typically manifested at the invocative level, that is, through the commanding voice of the super-ego.[8] In this case, the object *a* over-runs the subject in the form of a series of interrupted imperatives. On the one hand, Lacan considers these commandments as a direct manifestation of the Other's desire and of the lack in the Other as a signifying entity. On the other hand, the senseless imperatives imply a modeling of and a solution to the overwhelming desire of the Other, and the anxiety this desire implies. The guilt feelings that result from the super-ego's commandments bind the *jouissance* that would otherwise end up in anxiety.

Lacan (1962–63) situates the Ego-Ideal – "that part of the Other that is most convenient to introject" (p. 333) – at the level of dismay. The Ego-Ideal is a trait of the Other that orients the ego and from which ideal images take shape: ideal egos (cf. Lacan's double mirror). Looking at oneself from the position of the Ego-Ideal affirms the ego's power. In this context, the voice as object *a* accompanies the signifier at the level of the ideal. The cruelty of the super-ego in depression, in comparison, begins with dissociation from the Ego-Ideal. The super-ego's activity typically consists of playing the Ego-Ideal against the ego, which ends up in a confirmation of the subject's impotence.

Preliminary work in depressive experiences: rehabilitating the Other

Starting psychoanalytic work when in the grips of depressive complaints is a precarious business. For analysis to occur, a shift in the stagnation at the level of the Other is necessary, such that the articulation of the subject comes to the fore again. Often, this pre-supposes an active and somewhat challenging role by the analyst during the period preliminary to psychoanalysis proper. In this last section, we will elaborate on this idea by referring back to Lacan's own clinical practice.

A preliminary issue to address, prior to any treatment, is the subject's disinterest in seeking a solution for distress through the Other. This is a common problem among patients with depression – after all, dissociation from the Other is its core characteristic. Those who do address an analyst often have only a vague demand and frequently their consultation is merely an attempt to placate their family or friends. Typically, their speech is empty, and they are overwhelmed by depressive feelings. In these cases, preliminary work first consists of installing a working relationship, whereby the analyst's belief in the power of speech and analytic sessions is communicated. In order to establish a basis for further sessions, the importance of addressing painful issues with words that aim to articulate this pain must be symbolically recognized. This is only possible if the analyst explicitly manifests a desire to engage in analytic work and listens attentively to the analysand's speech. The French psychoanalyst Jean Clavreul, who was in analysis with Lacan, indicates that this is exactly what Lacan did in his case: "Lacan did not focus on my being full of difficulties or my being full of hope, he was only interested in what I said" (cf. Weill *et al.*, 2001, p. 31, my translation). The focus is not on Clavreul's psychological experiences, but *on his actual articulation of difficulties*. When Clavreul was hospitalized, shortly after the sessions started, Lacan visited him in the hospital some 20 times so that the analytic sessions could continue. By doing this, Lacan clearly demonstrated his investment in making sure that this difficult work of articulation would not stop.

Gérard Haddad, who also referred himself to Lacan because of his depressive complaints (cf. 2002, p. 18, 32, 43, 67), calls attention to Lacan's meticulous listening and his respect for the analysand's speech. Haddad recalls Lacan's warmth during the first sessions and relates that Lacan explicitly expressed his desire to work with him. For example, when he called Lacan after an early interruption of the sessions because of business travel, Lacan was quite insisting: "okay, we start tomorrow, *because we have to*".

Installing such process of full speech is not without difficulty. The struggle with depressive complaints often implies a tendency to interpret the analyst's discursive position as an object *a*, which always implies a lack at the level of the signifier, and in an imaginary way. Hence, the risk that silences and a premature switch to using the couch are interpreted as signs of disinterest by the analyst or as confirmation of the subject's despair. In this context, the message to be conveyed is that the symbolic Other is the grounding of the subject. This gives the analyst the duty of being present in such a way that the articulation of what moves the body is facilitated.

Preliminary conversations aim to produce what Lacan (1991b, p. 35, 37) calls 'hysterization', the act of addressing oneself to an Other because a problem had produced discontent. The start of analysis requires that the analysand-to-be must come to believe that his/her problem is symptomatic and that it contains sense and truth (cf. Lacan 1974–75). This implies a change in attitude towards one's problems since depressive phenomena typically overrun the subject and imply the position of a passive observer who remains paralyzed in relation to overwhelming issues (Vanheule, 2016). The analysts' preliminary interventions will have to confront this stagnation at the level of the Other and will consist of attempts at signifying discontent. The analyst should aim for a revitalization (cf. Kristeva, 1993) and re-metaphorization of language, whereby signifiers are linked to the Real of e-motion, of being moved. This means that the analyst has to effectively facilitate the naming of discontent and stimulate the analysand-to-be by elaborating the named discontent associatively. Such *naming*, and its associative elaboration, contradict the listlessness, and the apathy towards the articulation of depressive experiences.

This process of naming is clinically illustrated in the books of the psychoanalysts Catherine Millot (2001) and Gérard Haddad (2002), who were both in analysis with Lacan.

Millot consulted Lacan because of a problem she describes as a permanent confused state of emptiness and inhibition, mixed with anxiety, and a preoccupation with death. Lacan reacts to her descriptions by offering a signifier that closely connects to the chain of signifiers that she had already used: "Lacan answered me in the register of philosophy – that is of mysticism, where, for the lack of anything better, I had already been looking for my bearings" (Millot, 2001, p. 16). Lacan said the problem she described to him was "*Gelassenheit*" (literally: stillness, composure or serenity), a concept he borrowed from the German mystic Master Eckhart, whose oeuvre Millot was then reading intensely (Millot, 2001, p. 16). As she told him about her most negative experiences, he reacted by stating: "What you met there, is love" (Millot, 2001, p. 16). Later on, as she was brooding about a difficult issue in her life, he reacted by stating: "no one is expected to achieve the impossible" (Millot, 2001, p. 17). These reactions both confused her (i.e., tore her away from an empty discourse) and gave her an anchoring point within the domain of signifiers to proceed: "by naming it he gave legitimacy to that what seemed unacceptable" (Millot, 2001, p. 17).

When Haddad entered his analysis, he struggled with temporal disorientation and, more specifically, with the preoccupation of being too late. When he acted out this idea in one of the first sessions and claimed that he started analysis too late, that he was born too late, and that he felt saddened by it, Lacan reacted by saying that this feeling was a characteristic of his structure and that they would have to return to it. As Lacan closed the session he added: "One never encounters psychoanalysis too late" (Haddad, 2002, p. 99). This utterance confused Haddad but also stimulated him to continue the attempt of articulating his problems by means of the signifier: "It functioned like a clean sweep in my inhibitions; the support that subsequently allowed me to engage in the mad mission that I was still ignoring, meaning that I had actually asked to start an analysis" (Haddad, 2002, p. 99). By formulating such a hopeful claim that actually contradicted a central tenet that Haddad held on to, Lacan produced a transformation: depressive stagnation gets transformed into creative exploration.

On the basis of the table developed in Seminar X, we can say that the act of challenging stagnation aims at changing the subjective status of inhibitions, emotion, and dismay. By providing active support in articulating difficulties, facilitating the naming of discontent, and being present with a clear desire to engage in full speech, the analyst offers an anchoring point in the Other, and indeed, an anchoring point within the analysis itself, which impels the subject to take up the work of articulation through the signifier. This shift implies that the symptomatic value of inhibitions, emotion, and dismay is recognized. In Seminar X, Lacan (1962–63) describes inhibition as follows: "to be inhibited is a symptom tucked away in a museum" (p. 10). It is a potential symptom that is taken out of circulation at the level of the Other. Naming aims at the exact opposite, at bringing about the association of signifiers linked to the excluded element. As such, we argue that through symbolic naming, the subject is turned away from the left column towards the central category of the table – i.e., the symptom – which is the point at which psychoanalysis proper can start.

Notes

1　Lacan doesn't refer much to the work of these contemporaries. In 'propos sur la causalité psychique' (1946), he criticizes Ey's organo-dynamism – his attempt to make a parallel between dynamic mental factors and an organic substrate. In a review of Minkowski's book, 'Le temps vécu', Lacan (1935) criticizes the latter's phenomenological approach.

2　For example, in his review of Minkowski's 'Le temps vécu' Lacan (1935, p. 431, my translation) indicates the following about Minkowski's descriptions: "The only thing that seems most fundamental … is the subduction of experienced time in depressive states".

3　Throughout the Seminar Lacan frequently uses the concept 'phenomena' to indicate the clinical categories he introduces.

4　Lacan introduces this matrix in the beginning of Seminar X and returns to it at the end. This schema was never used in his writings and is little referred to in his later seminars. I don't agree with the explanation Hassoun (1995) gives of these two dimensions. He claims the three stages in both dimensions indicate, respectively, the imaginary, the symbolic and the real, but this interpretation is not rooted in the context of the tenth seminar. In his book on Seminar X, Harari (2001) unfortunately doesn't address in sufficient depth the precise meaning of both dimensions, nor does Razavet (2000) in his comments on Seminar X.

5　In his comments on 'Inhibitions, Symptoms and Anxiety' Miller (1997-98, 19 November 1997) links the idea of movement to the Freudian pleasure principle. In line with Lacan's comments on that text, Miller, too, discerns two dimensions at work: the dimension of fiction and the signifier on the one hand, and on the other the dimension of the Real and the drive (cf. Miller, 1997-98, 19 November 1997, 10 December 1997).

6 Here Lacan is referring explicitly to Dante's 'Divine Comedy', where in the 'Inferno' volume (Canto 30, line 139-144), Dante makes a direct link between not having spoken and sadness.

7 In hysterical neurosis, dismay will primarily manifest itself at the oral level. This can be observed in Freud's case of Katharina, who reacts to her primal scene with the following reaction: "My throat is squeezed together as though I were going to choke" (Freud, 1895, p. 126).

8 See also Lacan's Graph, where he situates the super-ego at the level of the voice; beyond the realm of the Other (Lacan, 1991a).

References

Allen, D.F. (2001). Lacan aurait cent ans. *Evolution psychiatrique*, *66*, 199–202.

Angst, J. (1997). Epidemiology of depression. In A. Honig & H.M. Van Praag (Eds.), *Depression*. New York: John Wiley.

Ehrenberg, A. (1998). *La fatigue d'être soi: Dépression et société*. Paris: Odile Jacob.

Ey, H. (1954). *Etudes psychiatriques*. Paris: Desclee de Brouwer.

Ey, H., Bernard, P., & Brisset, Ch. (1967). *Manuel de psychiatrie (3e edition)*. Paris: Masson.

Freud, S. (1895). Studies in hysteria. In J. Strachey (Ed.), *The Standard Edition of the Complete Psychological Works of Sigmund Freud*, Volume II. London: Hogarth Press.

Freud, S. (1915). Instincts and their vicissitudes. In J. Strachey (Ed.), *The Standard Edition of the Complete Psychological Works of Sigmund Freud*, Volume XIV (pp. 109–140). London: Hogarth Press.

Freud, S. (1926). Inhibitions, symptoms and anxiety. In J. Strachey (Ed.), *The Standard Edition of the Complete Psychological Works of Sigmund Freud, Volume XX* (pp. 77–175). London: Hogarth Press.

Freud, S. (1933). New introductory lectures onpPsycho-analysis. In J. Strachey (Ed.), *The Standard Edition of the Complete Psychological Works of Sigmund Freud*, Volume XXII. London: Hogarth Press.

Fuchs, T. (2001). Melancholia as a desynchronization. Towards a psychopathology of interpersonal time. *Psychopathology*, *34*, 179–186.

Haddad, G. (2002). *Le jour où Lacan m'a adopté*. Paris: Grasset.

Harari, R. (2001). *Lacan's Seminar on "Anxiety", an Introduction*. New York: Other Press.

Hassoun, J. (1995). *La cruauté mélancholique*. Paris: Aubier.

Kristeva, J. (1993). *Les nouvelles maladies de l'âme*. Paris: Fayard.

Lacan, J. (1935). Compte rendu de E. Minkowski 'Le Temps vécu. Etudes phénoménologiques et psychologiqes'. *Recherches Philosophiques*, *5*, 424–431.

Lacan, J. (1946). Propos sur la causalité psychique. *Ecrits* (pp. 151–193). Paris: Seuil.

Lacan, J (1962–1963). *The Seminar, Book X, Anxiety*. Cambridge & Malden: Polity, 2014.

Lacan, J. (1964–1965). *Le Séminaire XII, Problèmes cruciaux pour la psychanalyse*. Unpublished.

Lacan, J. (1965). La science et la vérité. *Ecrits* (pp. 855–877). Paris: Seuil.

Lacan, J. (1973). *Le Séminaire, Livre XI, Les quatre concepts fondamentaux de la psychanalyse*. J.A. Miller (Ed.). Paris: Seuil.

Lacan, J. (1974–1975). *Le Séminaire XXII, RSI*. Unpublished.

Lacan, J. (1975). Intervention dans la séance de travail « Sur la passe » du samedi 3 novembre 1973. *Lettres de l'Ecole freudienne, 15*, 185–193.

Lacan, J. (1990). *Television.* New York & London: Norton. (Original work published 1974)

Lacan, J. (1991a). *Le Séminaire, Livre VIII, Le transfert.* J.-A. Miller (Ed.). Paris: Seuil.

Lacan, J. (1991b). *Le Séminaire, Livre XVII, L'envers de la psychanalyse.* J.-A. Miller (Ed.). Paris: Seuil.

Lacan, J. (1994). *Le Séminaire, Livre IV, La relation d'objet.* J.-A. Miller (Ed.). Paris: Seuil.

Lepine, J.P., Gastpar, M., Mendlewicz, J., & Tylee, A. (1997). Depression in the community: the first pan-European study DEPRES (Depression Research in European Society). *International Journal of Clinical Psychopharmacology, 12*, 19–29.

Miller, J.-A. (1996–1997). *L'Autre qui n'existe pas et ses comités d'éthique.* Unpublished seminar.

Miller, J.-A. (1997–1998). *Le partenaire-symptôme.* Unpublished seminar.

Millot, C. (2001). *Abîmes Ordinaries.* Paris: Gallimard.

Minkowski, E. (1933). *Le temps vécu.* Paris: d'artey.

Razavet, J.-C. (2000). *De Freud à Lacan. De roc de la castration au roc de la structure.* Paris: De Boeck.

Smith, R. (1992). *Inhibition: History and Meaning in the Sciences of Mind and Brain.* London: Free Association Books.

Vanheule, S. (2001). Inhibition: 'I am because I don't act'. *The Letter, 23*, 109–126.

Vanheule, S. (2016). Capitalist discourse, subjectivity and Lacanian Psychoanalysis. *Frontiers in Psychology, 7*, 1948. doi: 10.3389/fpsyg.2016.01948.

Weill, A.D., Weiss, E., & Gravas, F. (2001). *Quartier Lacan.* Paris: Denoël.

Widlöcher, D. (1995). *Les logiques de la depression.* Paris: Fayard.

Chapter 3

Forgetting and remembering

Russell Grigg

What is mourning? What is it, really, that a person goes through when he or she loses someone they love … I mean really loves? And another question. What is it to mourn no longer? What state does the person who has loved and lost find themselves in 'at the end,' when they have finally overcome their grief? When one can 'get on with one's life,' as they say? Is it that one has got over one's loss? In a sense, yes, of course, one has gotten over one's loss. But, if this means that one has forgotten the person one has lost, then, no, the lost loved one is not forgotten. Even as the pain of loss diminishes, so the memory remains.

What I argue is that, at the end of grieving, the lost person is not forgotten but commemorated. And it's this commemoration that I want to speak of.

Freud says something very odd about mourning in his classic paper on the topic. You know the thesis: in mourning, each of the memories in which the libido is bound to the object is brought up and hypercathected, so that the libido can detach itself from it and the ego can be "free and uninhibited again" at the end of the process (Freud, 1917, p. 245). I've argued against this claim: it is such a manifestly untrue remark that I find it curious that Freud should have made it. It is obvious to the most casual observer that mourning always leaves traces behind, in the form of often painful memories of a loved one. Even though the pain of the memories dulls with time, they remain liable to resurface at special moments such as anniversaries, just as they can also emerge in connection with the most unexpected things: a movie, an item of clothing, a memory of a holiday, or even with a new love. A lost object rarely disappears entirely; an object that was once loved and lost is probably never abandoned without a trace. And yet, according to Freud, mourning involves a process of abandonment of one's attachment to the memories of the lost object, and, as slow and painful as this process may be, there will be a return to the status *quo ante*. In the "normal case," he says, there is a withdrawal of the libido invested in the object and a reassignment to a new one. It is only in the pathological case of melancholia that the lost object remains, where, as he says, "the shadow of the object fell upon the ego" (Freud, 1917, p. 249). But, even in normal mourning, the lost object always casts its shadow upon the ego. Even if it is true that the normal process of mourning is over when one is free of

DOI: 10.4324/9781003216391-4

the object's hold and can live and love again, the ego never completely loses the mark of the object that has been lost.

As it turns out, Freud does recognize that a lost love object is, in fact, never completely abandoned and remains irreplaceable. Strangely, it took the tragic death in 1920 of Freud's fifth child, Sophie, at the age of 26, from Spanish influenza, for Freud to realize this. Indeed, he recognized that the reason for the continued attachment to the object that keeps the object alive – that memorializes it, as it were – is the very love for the object itself. On February 4th of that same year, 1920, he wrote to Ferenczi of his "insurmountable narcissistic insult" (Freud & Ferenczi, 1920–1933, p. 7). Then, some nine years later on April 11, 1929, in a letter consoling Ludwig Binswanger who had undergone a similar loss, Freud wrote,

> We know that the acute sorrow we feel after such a loss will run its course, but also that we will remain inconsolable, and will never find a substitute. No matter what may come to take its place, even should it fill that place completely, it remains something else. *And that is how it should be.* It is the only way of perpetuating a love that we do not want to abandon.
>
> (Freud & Binswanger, 1908–1938, p. 196)

"And that is how it should be," writes Freud. The mourning does not and should not bring an end to the object's presence in one's life. The process of mourning a lost object can go hand in hand with a persistent drive to memorialize the lost person and one's relationship to him or her. It is as if, out of respect for the person and one's attachment to him or her, one is bent on maintaining the memory of one's attachment to the object so that the object itself somehow outlives the psychical work of mourning. This commemoration, carrying the memory of others, is a fundamental feature of mourning and loss. As Goethe is said to have written, "We die twice: first when we die and then when those who knew and loved us die," and it is as living memorials that we carry the mark of lost loved ones on our souls.

When the mourning is over, the object is still preserved in some way; *and this is as it should be.* As more or less distressful as the persistent memory of a lost loved one may be, there may be no question for the person who has suffered a loss of ever wanting to forget that loss. Moreover, the sadness, regret, and pain experienced over a loss can be experienced without having any impact on the person's self-regard. One's life may be impoverished by the loss of a loved one, but without one's sense of one's worth being diminished.

Mourning gives expression to an important push to memorialization as an expression of respect for the dead demanded of and by the bereaved, those who loved and have, in a sense, been left behind by the death of a friend or loved one.

Julian Barnes gives eloquent expression to the dilemma of the griever: What is 'success' in mourning, he asks? Does it lie in remembering or in forgetting?

Clearly, the griever sees their mourning in moral terms. When we mourn, we are not just narcissistically pained by our loss, which is the "narcissistic wound"

Freud refers to, but we also have a moral attachment – a commitment if you will – to the memory of the person who has gone. What sort of commitment is it? Well, as we say, we have a commitment to their memory. We have a commitment to memorializing the object we have loved, and this memorialization requires an inscription, of some kind, in the symbolic. The memorialization of what is lost entails leaving a record in the Other, the symbolic, of the object's disappearance. And, because it is registered in the Other, it is crucial that this record be both public and private, both material and psychical. Mourning is every bit as much about public ritual and commemoration as about internal psychical work.

While there are obvious narcissistic components to the process of mourning, where the mourner can become self-obsessed and fixated on his loss, we judge this morally. Again, I quote Barnes (2013, 113):

Look how much I loved him/her and with these my tears I prove it.
    Look how much I suffer, how much others fail to understand: does this not prove how much I loved?
    Maybe, maybe not.

I have proposed that mourning is not so much about forgetting as it is about remembering. We can now add that mourning seems to be about finding the right way to remember. Or, as I would prefer, the right way to commemorate.

The rituals of mourning are part of, are essential to, the 'right' way to commemorate. The rituals of mourning are so important that the noun 'mourner' does not refer to a person's grief, or at least does so only indirectly. A 'mourner' is first and foremost someone performing a ritual. She is someone who attends a funeral or who is said to be 'in mourning,' frequently in a way that is prescribed either by religious law or popular custom. Mourning can mean wearing black; it can last for two weeks or 40 days, where the period of mourning is frequently calculated to the day. In some cultures, it is even possible to employ professional mourners to make a public demonstration of grief to honor the deceased. In any case, the practice of mourning is less an indication of the extent of a person's grief than a ritual that is more or less correctly carried out as a mark of respect for the deceased. Again, even where the practice of mourning is not clearly circumscribed, there are still considerations of propriety that bear on the activities associated with mourning. As Hamlet sarcastically puts it, "Thrift, thrift, Horatio! The funeral baked meats / Did coldly furnish forth the marriage tables" (Shakespeare 1.2.179–180).

But what about the internal work of mourning, the psychical work that a griever undergoes? How are we to understand the psychical process of mourning? Freud's account won't do because it is about forgetting, withdrawal of cathexis, and reinvestment in a new object – a view which he subsequently abandons, even if only implicitly when he refers to the death of his daughter Sophie, and the ethical requirement not to forget.

Let's think about mourning in terms of memorializing. First, it needs to be based on memorializing in the right way. As Lacan says in the discussion of Hamlet in Désir et Son Interprétation (*Seminar VI, Desire and Its Interpretation*), Hamlet's father is not yet dead and walks the stage restlessly at night precisely because he has not been properly memorialized – where, in an era when the values of honor and nobility prevailed, avenging his murder was essential to proper memorialization. I'll come back to this question of the 'right way.' For the moment, let's say something about the mechanism of mourning.

In Chapter 18 of *Seminar VI*, "Mourning and Desire," Lacan briefly comments that mourning is like the inverse of *Verwerfung*. More precisely, he says that with the grief over the loss of a loved one, a hole opens up in the real such that the subject enters into a relationship that is the "converse of … *Verwerfung*." Clarifying this, Lacan (2019) adds that this hole in the Real "sets in motion … the signifier that can only be purchased with your own flesh and your own blood, the signifier that is essentially the veiled phallus" (p. 336, translation modified). The suggestion here, then, seems to be that the breach in reality created by the loss of a loved one sets in train, in the reverse direction, the process typically involved in the triggering of a psychosis. Instead of the calamitous collapse, as in psychosis, of signifiers that reveal the absence of the Name-of-the-Father, in mourning the loss unconsciously activates afresh phallic signifiers that libidinally bind one to the love object. This explains why, in mourning, the memories of the lost object become so vivid, why everything reminds one of the lost object, or why it fills one's dreams. Thus, whereas Freud took the approach that the work of mourning is a process of relinquishing the features of the object one by one, slowly and painstakingly, Lacan here regards the process as one of the preservation of the object by constructing a memorial to it in the symbolic.

I think that the mechanism of mourning looks more or less like this: the work of mourning consists of codifying imaginary features of the object, *i(a)*, into signifiers lodged in the Other. The painful process of mourning stems from the fall of the semblants that love and desire attach us to, as Freud taught us; but – and this is what Freud did not capture – the work of mourning is the transformation of these semblants into signifiers registered in and endorsed by the Other. It is the combination of ritual as a community event – funerals, mourning practices, etc. – with the individual's psychical work of mourning that achieves this commemoration. Identification with the lost object, or rather with traits of the lost object, is a part and part only of this process.

This is not the whole story about mourning, which also contains a real dimension involving the subject's relation to the object *a*. In mourning, the painful loss of one's semblants exposes the underlying object *a*, the cause of one's desire, and the object that one has put in place to support one's castration. This is the exposure to the real of the object *a*, or at least a particular aspect of it, which is ordinarily hidden by the object's ideal features. Hidden in mourning, but manifest in melancholia.

We are familiar with this process in our analytic experience where the end of analysis is akin to this process, albeit in attenuated form. This is the 'slow burn' that constitutes analysis, which I have spoken about elsewhere. Melanie Klein recognized this as a form of mourning. Recasting Klein, it is possible, then, to think of the progress of analysis as a sort of non-traumatic traumatization, or, if you wish, as a controlled decline of the imaginary. In analysis, the fall of semblants results, not from the slings and arrows of misfortune; rather, the fall of semblants results, slowly, and in a way regulated by interpretation, from the analysis itself. This of course makes analysis a process that has less to do with the healing of wounds, the recuperation of the subject's identity, or a return to the status quo ante in such cases. Interpretation, and indeed the process of analysis itself, is a less brutal means of dissolving the artifacts with which the individual's narcissism is surrounded. And a gentle awakening, a slow trauma, as when we say a 'slow burn,' that is calculated and ratified by the subject, is undoubtedly more beneficial than the unforeseen crisis apt to result from the sadism or cynicism of the Other.

Incidentally, this is where the essential difference between melancholia and mourning lies. In the exposure to the real of the object a, the melancholic subject turns out to be defenseless against the object. The object cannot be memorialized, as it can be in mourning, but instead remains there forever in the real. The collapse of semblants that otherwise veil the object persists, and the 'grimace' of the object, like the grimace of a skull behind a beautiful face, is exposed; for the melancholic, the veil of semblants, the $i(a)$, over the object a falls altogether.

Can we understand melancholia as a psychotic process? I believe so. An account might look something like this. The symbolic order regulates imaginary *jouissance*, subtracting it from the subject in the process. This subtraction of *jouissance*, which we write as $(-\varphi)$, takes place at the level of libido and the drive. Now, because in psychosis the Name-of-the-Father is foreclosed, the possibility opens of an excess of imaginary *jouissance* that is both unregulated and invasive. The disarray and confusion that Schreber, for instance, initially finds himself in are accompanied by invasive imaginary *jouissance*. Then, over the course of his psychosis, he discovers a new way of regulating his *jouissance*, which involves constructing a new relationship with the world, which emerges with his delusional metaphor.

The stability of Schreber's paranoid delusion contrasts with the earlier phase of the disorder when the excess of *jouissance* simply overwhelms him. In his "On a Question Prior to Any Possible Treatment of Psychosis," Lacan (2006) describes the early confusional period of the psychosis as the "subject's regression – a topographical, not a genetic, regression – to the mirror stage," wherein the relationship to "the specular other is reduced here to its mortal impact" (p. 473). Schreber's voices, for instance, speak of him as a "leper corpse leading another leper corpse", and his body as merely "an aggregate of colonies of foreign 'nerves,' a sort of dump for detached fragments of his persecutors' identities" (p. 473). Lacan's analysis is in terms of the distinction between the imaginary and the symbolic. The mortification in question is the result of the structural regression to the imaginary relationship. The object in the real plays no part.

One could speculate that if Lacan had written this text post-1964 instead of in 1958, he would have invoked the role object *a* has to play. He would have referred the mortiferous role to the object, not to a regression to the imaginary. And he would have distinguished between the collapse of phallic signification, "Φ_0," in Schema I, and the unmediated presence of object *a*. In a 1967 address by Lacan to a meeting of psychiatrists at the Sainte Anne Hospital, as part of a series of lectures under the auspices of his friend Henri Ey, we find this comment:

> It is the free men, the truly free men, who are mad. There is no demand for the petit *a*, he holds it, it is what he calls his voices, for instance. [...] He does not cling to the locus of the Other, the big Other, through the object *a*, he has it at his disposal. [...] Let's say that he has his cause in his pocket, and that is why he is mad.
>
> (Lacan, 1967, p. 10)

The proximity of the object *a* in psychosis means that the subject has not separated himself from it as the object cause of desire. This separation, which for the neurotic subject is produced by the Other as the locus of speech and language, both regulates and limits his *jouissance*. In the absence of this separation a plenitude of *jouissance* is apparent in such typical psychotic formations as erotomania, hypochondriasis, and the persecutions characteristic of paranoia, as well as the feminization of the psychotic subject, or what Lacan calls the '*pousse-à-la-femme*' we find in many transsexuals, with their unbridgeable certainty and the sometimes persistent pursuit of surgical interventions to better approximate their resemblance to their particular ideal of femininity.

In melancholia, we encounter the same failure of separation from the object. The depressive function is explained by the fact that the unseparated-off object, in being a 'piece of the real,' ('*un bout de réel*,' as Lacan says) leaves the subject exposed and defenseless to its ravages. A comparison with paranoia might help: the paranoiac is prey to the evil Other who wishes him ill; the melancholic is likewise defenseless against the real of a horrific object, unmediated by the symbolic.

Lacan talks of melancholia very rarely and does not offer much of an account of affective or passional psychoses, despite Clérambault's attention to it. I think we can understand melancholia in these terms: while the neurotic's access to a libidinal object is *via* its semblants, in melancholia the veil of semblants falls from the object, leaving the melancholic exposed to the object in the real and at its mercy. This object can be either persecutory, as it is in paranoia, or abject-making, as in melancholia.

Thus, when Freud proceeds by comparing and contrasting mourning and melancholia, it is a little misleading. The melancholic suffers not from eternal mourning but from an inescapable proximity to the object in the real. In neurosis, there is a phallic presentation of the object and its semblants, while in melancholia the encounter with the real object is at stake.

To return to dreams and trauma after a long detour *via* the object in the real present in mourning and melancholia, let me refer you to Lacan's discussion of the dream reported by Freud in the *Traumdeutung*, "Father, don't you see I am burning." Lacan's genius is to demonstrate the traumatic element at the heart of the dream by taking the very example that Freud had given to illustrate the claim that dreams are the guardian of sleep. As Lacan demonstrates, at the heart of the primary process "we see preserved the insistence of the trauma in making us aware of its existence" (Lacan, 1977, p. 55). And then, "the reality system [...] leaves an essential part of what belongs to the real a prisoner in the web of the pleasure principle" (Lacan, 1977, p. 55). In this preservation of the insistence of the trauma, we can detect the link with memorialization that I have been arguing for, whether there in the dream's traumatic repetition, or there in the memorialization in mourning, or there in the failed memorialization of the object in melancholia.

References

Barnes, J. (2013). *Levels of Life*. New York: Random House.

Freud, S. (1917). Mourning and Melancholia. In J. Strachey (Ed.), *The Standard Edition of the Complete Psychological Works of Sigmund Freud*, Vol. XIV, 237–258. London: Hogarth Press.

Freud, S. & Binswanger, L. (1908–1938). *The Sigmund Freud-Ludwig Binswanger Correspondence, 1908–1938*. F. Gerhard (Ed.). (A. J. Pomerans, Trans.). London: Open Gate Press, 2003.

Freud, S. & Ferenczi, S. (1920–1933). *The Correspondence of Sigmund Freud and Sandor Ferenczi*, Vol. 3. E. Brabant, E. Falzeder, & P. Giampieri-Deutsch (Eds.). (P. T. Hoffer, Trans.). Cambridge, MA: Harvard University Press, 2000.

Lacan, J. (1967). La formation du psychiatre et la psychanalyse. *École lacanienne de psychanalyse*. Retrieved from www.ecole-lacanienne.net/documents/1967- 11-10.doc

Lacan, J. (1977). *Seminar XI: The Four Fundamental Concepts of Psycho-Analysis*. J. A. Miller (Ed.). (A. Sheridan, Trans.). London: The Hogarth Press.

Lacan, J. (2006). On a Question Prior to Any Possible Treatment of Psychosis. In *Écrits: The First Complete Edition in English*, 445–488. (B. Fink, Trans.). London: W. W. Norton & Company.

Lacan, J. (2019). *Desire and Its Interpretation, The Seminar VI*. J. A. Miller (Ed.). (B. Fink, Trans.). Cambridge: Polity, 2019.

Shakespeare, W. (1992). *Hamlet*. B. A. Mowat & P. Werstine (Eds.). New York: Simon Schuster.

Chapter 4

Some thoughts on Mourning and Melancholia

Darian Leader

Given the fact that many psychoanalysts claim that their work is all about allowing a patient to mourn some unresolved loss, it is remarkable how little psychoanalytic literature has been produced on the question of what exactly mourning consists of. Psychologists and psychologically minded psychoanalysts have provided fine descriptions of the phenomena involved in the grieving process while shying away from metapsychological accounts. Today, the prevalence of the motifs of mourning and grief in popular psychology has perhaps encouraged analysts to keep their distance even more resolutely.

Freud's classic account, 'Mourning and Melancholia', drafted in 1915 and published some two years later, was the first sustained psychoanalytic study of the processes that follow the experience of loss. His earlier hypotheses on melancholia, mostly contained in the letters he wrote to Wilhelm Fliess between 1887 and 1902, would remain largely unelaborated until the 1915 draft. After the publication of 'Mourning and Melancholia', Freud's comments on the issues involved are quite sparse: he returns to the question of the diversity of reactions following a loss in an appendix to 'Inhibition, Symptom, Anxiety', and he generalises his hypothesis on melancholic identification in 'The Ego and the Id'. For later historians of these notions, Freud's theory remained confined to the one seminal 1915 paper.

If we agree with most of its close readers that 'Mourning and Melancholia' contains a number of contradictions, unexplored questions, and suggestions for further research, it is especially curious that psychoanalytic writers have not expended more ink on the subject. Those analysts who have gone back to the themes of Freud's essay have, in fact, almost universally disagreed with him. The division between mourning and melancholia, for example, seemed too neat to many commentators, and the partitioning of criteria to characterise the two conditions alien to clinical experience. For example, it was remarked that so-called ambivalence was hardly confined to pathological mourning or melancholia and that bursts of manic behaviour and 'triumph' could certainly be found throughout the spectrum of grieving processes.

In the Lacanian tradition, the paucity of writing on mourning and melancholia is also noticeable. Lacan devoted a few sessions of his seminar to a discussion

DOI: 10.4324/9781003216391-5

of mourning, although in his written work the term only appears seven times (Allouch, 1995, p. 157). As for melancholia, there are three references in the written work and merely a handful in the seminars. To further an understanding of Lacan's views on melancholia, we would need the testimony of those who attended his clinical presentations where the diagnosis was occasionally made. Lacanians today recognise melancholia as a clinical category, but extended discussions are scarce, and its metapsychology tends to be reduced to aphorisms that are, for the most part, purely descriptive. Moreover, these often merely echo the symmetry searched for by late nineteenth-century psychiatry between paranoia on the one hand and melancholia on the other. Exceptions to this often cursory treatment are found in the series of works by Christian Vereecken (1986, 1993–1994), and, recently, in studies by Frédéric Pellion (2000) and Geneviève Morel (2002).

Although it is clear that a focus on the now popular notion of depression (and its subcategories) might render obsolete the study of an apparently andeluvian concept like melancholia, the lack of attention in Lacanian circles is still surprising given the current use of the diagnosis. As for mourning, the rarity of contributions to this question by students of Lacan seems congruent with the more general avoidance of the theme in analytic literature. Jean Allouch's (1995) recent study stands out as an exception here (see also Menard, 1982; Turnheim, 1997). One might argue, indeed, that mourning is, in fact, the province of literature rather than psychoanalysis. Yet the fact that literary fiction is a culture's privileged arena for the exploration of loss should in no way be an argument for its neglect by analytic commentators. In fact, quite the opposite.

Without attempting any kind of democratic survey of Freudian, Post-Freudian and Lacanian work on mourning and melancholia, I will examine Freud's 1915 paper and what are arguably the most significant analytic responses to it: those of Abraham, Klein and Lacan. After a selective discussion of Lacan's views on the mourning process, we will see how Klein and Lacan both seem to have been converging on particular aspects of mourning which can help us to situate the clinical phenomena with greater clarity. We will then move on to a more general discussion of mourning and melancholia and suggest some questions for further research.

'Mourning and Melancholia'

The many recent studies of the concept of melancholy tend to agree that Freud's 1915 paper was something of a landmark. These historical accounts have highlighted the shifting forms of melancholy and the instability of its characterising symptoms (Radden, 1987; Radden, 2000; Jackson, 1986). If any common and defining symptoms can be found, these were a sense of fear and sorrow without obvious cause. Until well into the nineteenth century, sadness and low affects were not defining features (Radden, 2000; Babb, 1951). Indeed, fixation on a single theme, later known as monomania, was a much more common criterion. Curiously, the clinical picture of melancholia that we can distil from such accounts puts a much greater emphasis on anxiety than on so-called depressive affects, a fact that is echoed in the history of biochemical responses (Healy, 1997).

In Freud's contribution, however, self-reproach and loss become crucial variables, and although this may seem obvious to us today, the link of melancholic states to the experience of loss had not been treated in such a systematic way before Freud. Reading earlier texts on melancholia, we come across occasional references to the power of bereavement to push the subject into melancholy, but these tend to be treated in the medical literature as contingent and rather episodic details. Although this may surprise us, we should be aware that the notion of 'loss' that we are familiar with today is probably a rather recent construction, with its roots in nineteenth-century Romanticism. Hence how it seems deeply conservative in terms of nineteenth-century notions of mourning, even though Freud's essay seems radical in terms of earlier theories of melancholia. Philippe Ariès, for example, saw 'Mourning and Melancholia' as one of the last great texts of the Romantic movement (Ariès, 1977; Allouch, 1995).

Whereas classical and premodern responses to bereavement involved formalised public displays and the involvement of the community, the mourning described by Freud is an intensely private process. The individual is alone with their mourning. Indeed, there are no references in his discussion to the participation of other people in the process of grieving, a feature that has continually surprised commentators on Freud's text. Geoffrey Gorer (1965) drew attention to this in his influential survey 'Death, Grief and Mourning', pointing out that every documented human society has mourning rituals that involve public displays of some sort. Gorer, and others, have argued that the decline of public mourning must be linked to the mass slaughter of the First World War and the radical changes that this introduced in societal responses to death (Capdevila & Voldman, 2002).

It was during this period of the redrafting of bereavement ritual that Freud began his text on mourning and melancholia. He is careful to state at the opening of his discussion that it never occurs to anyone to regard mourning as a pathological condition, although, if we take mourning to refer to its outward manifestations, this is arguably exactly the process that was taking place at the time that Freud penned his article (Gorer 1965). For Freud, mourning involves the long and painful work of detaching the libido from its object. Each memory and expectation linked to the object must be brought up and the libido detached from it, although Freud (1917) notes that this piecemeal process prolongs psychically the existence of the lost object (p. 245). The judgement that the object no longer exists resulting from this process is termed by Freud as 'reality testing' or 'proving' (Realitätsprüfung), suggesting that access to 'reality' is based on the registration of loss.

Freud's expository section on mourning thus raises a rather tricky question: if moving through all the details, memories and expectations linked to the object prolongs its existence, how can this be reconciled with the idea that this process results in a detachment from the object? Does something further have to take place? Is there a moment in the process when the existence of the object slides into non-existence? Freud's formulation might seem to imply that there will be a moment when all aspects of the attachment to the object will be run through, and the prolonged existence severed. This is a question we will come back to later on, and it suggests that, beyond the actual 'work' of mourning described by Freud, something has to happen to the work of mourning itself.

The focus on memories and expectations linked to the lost object involved in mourning will concern the dynamic of word and thing representations, a theme that is central throughout the metapsychological papers. In 'Mourning and Melancholia', the assumption seems to be something like this: mourning can be carried out due to the possibility of movement from thing representations to word representations. The operator here is the system Preconscious, which enables a passage from one representational system to another. As each aspect of the thing representation is made subject to the judgements of mourning, the affects linked to it are fractioned in what Freud calls a 'detail work'. The fact that the object must be accessed in all its different registrations in these systems implies that mourning will be a long and painful process.

The melancholic picture is different. Freud argues that a barrier prevents the usual passage between systems of representation. Unconscious thing representations cannot be accessed through word representations, as the path *via* the system Preconscious is blocked. The subject is left in the limbo of the impossible passage from one to the other. These considerations tend to be eclipsed by what Freud has to say about melancholia's characteristic self-reproach. Although it shares with mourning such features as "a profoundly painful dejection, cessation of interest in the outside world, loss of the capacity to love" and inhibition of activity, its prime distinguishing trait is "a lowering of self-regarding feelings to a degree that finds utterance in self-reproaches and self-revilings, and culminates in a delusional expectation of punishment" (Freud, 1917, p. 244). The melancholic represents his ego as "poor, worthless and despicable, and expects to be cast out and punished" (p. 246). These self-reproaches concern the very being of the subject, and thus differ from the feelings of lack of self-worth that we might find in other clinical structures where the emphasis is on the inadequacy of the body image (p. 248).

Pursuing the contrast with mourning, Freud argues that while the mourner knows more or less what has been lost, this is not always obvious to the melancholic subject. The nature of the object loss is not necessarily conscious and may just as well involve a disappointment or slight from the object as the loss occasioned by bereavement. And, if the melancholic does have an idea of whom he has lost, he does not know, Freud (1917) says, "what he has lost" in them (p. 245). This latter remark is crucial to situate not only Freud's views on melancholia but also those of Lacan that would follow: it implies, after all, that there is a difference between a 'who' and a 'what' in the field of loss, a theme we will return to later in our discussion.

Most of the later commentaries on the 1917 text see self-reproach, rather than the relations between the systems of representations, as Freud's key differential marker between mourning and melancholia. And certainly, self-reproach not only has a central place in the discussion but also in his earlier formulations of psychic life. Note first of all a problem with translation. Where the English text distinguishes frequently between 'reproach' and 'self-reproach', Freud's German does so much less frequently. Freud's term 'Vorwurf' (reproach) is translated as both 'reproach' and 'self-reproach' depending on how the translators saw fit. Bearing this in mind, we can cast an eye over this concept that Freud had called, in an 1899 letter to Fliess, "truly a neglected corner of psychic life" (Freud, 1985, p. 390).

In the Fliess letters and drafts, we find the major clinical structures linked to modalities of the subject's relation to the category of self-reproach. In the sequence that Freud posits for the genesis of obsession, for example, an early experience of pleasure is followed by self-reproach. Both of these are subsequently repressed, to leave a vague sense of guilt. In paranoia, the reproach is projected outside the subject, to maintain the conviction of the paranoiac's innocence (Freud, 1985, pp. 164–167). With hysteria, Freud mentions the possibility of self-reproaches due to death wishes directed to a loved one, an idea that he returns to many years later in his study of Dostoevsky. A further model present in the Fliess letters, although largely unelaborated, concerns self-reproach *via* identification with a woman of low morals "in sexual connection with father or brother" (p. 241).

This last reference to identification is no doubt music to Lacanian ears as it supposes already a triangular model of hysteria: it is not just that the subject identifies with a woman of low morals, but that this identification is predicated on the place of that woman in the desire of a third party – i.e., the father or brother. On a more general level, we can make two points about the notion of self-reproach in the Fliess letters and drafts. First, in these early formulations, self-reproach is a primary position of the subject in relation to libidinal excitation and desire. It functions like a first judgement. Second, we should distinguish self-reproach as a question about sexuality from self-reproach as a response: the triangular model of hysteria may include self-reproach as part of a questioning process, whereas melancholia involves a fixity well-known to Freud and his predecessors. Trying to persuade a melancholic subject that their self-reproach was unjustified seemed fruitless to Freud and the authors of medical textbooks written long before 'Mourning and Melancholia'.

How does Freud explain the predominance of self-reproach in the 1915 text? Freud's hypothesis here is the exact opposite of that of Samuel Butler, who, in his 'Characters' of 1659, claimed that "A melancholic man is one that keeps the worst company in the world, that is, his own". Freud, on the contrary, argues that the company kept by the melancholic is rather that of his object, which has been drawn into the ego. The clamorous self-reproaches are, in fact, reproaches directed to a loved object that has been shifted onto the ego (Freud, 1917, p. 248). This may be someone the subject loves or has loved, or even should have loved, and, once transferred in this way, the ego is now judged as if it were the forsaken object. In Freud's famous phrase, "the shadow of the object" has fallen on the ego, now subject to the merciless criticism so singular to the melancholic subject.

Given the well-documented prevalence of such criticism and the auditory core of the superego emphasised by Lacan, we might wonder why it is that auditory hallucinations are relatively rare in melancholia.

Freud is careful to distinguish between the question of object cathexis and that of the object as such. Identification with the lost object takes the place of the initial object attachment. After some slight or disappointment, the object cathexis is brought to an end, and rather than a new object choice being made, the libido withdraws into the ego in the identification with the abandoned object. Freud notes the apparent contradiction here: how can it be so easy to renounce an object cathexis given what appears to be an initially strong attachment to the object? The answer, which Freud attributes to Rank, lies in the fact that the object choice was narcissistic. When the object cathexis is blocked, there is therefore a regression to narcissism (Freud, 1917, p. 249). What this means is that the love relation is not given up: narcissistic identification is a 'substitute' (Ersatz) here for erotic cathexis.

As Freud would put it in his correspondence with Ferenczi, love for the object cannot be given up even if the object is. Instead, this love takes refuge in narcissism (Freud, 1996, pp. 47–48). Part of the erotic cathexis of the object regresses to identification, while the other part – and this is crucial for the question of self-reproach – is involved in hating the object. We remember that the subject had suffered a slight or disappointment or neglect from the object, and the responses to this will be brought into play in the attacks on the subject's ego, newly minted with the shadow of the object. Contrary to many hasty readings of Freud's text here, he does not make hatred or ambivalence specific to melancholia. What he does is show how this hatred may be drawn into the service of the melancholic's narcissistic conflict to account for the phenomenon of self-reproach.

In obsessional neurosis, hostile feelings towards the object are quite usual, Freud notes, and they tend to give a "pathological cast" to the mourning process. The subject can reproach himself for the death of the object but in a way quite different from melancholia in the sense that there isn't any regressive drawing in of libido. In such instances, we are dealing with 'pathological mourning' but still not melancholia as such (Freud, 1917, p. 250). As for the sources of the hatred itself, Freud thinks that it is due to real experiences and constitutional factors, although he is reserved about what these may consist of. We should remember that by 'constitutional', Freud simply means psychically structured, in the sense of "elements of every love relation formed by that particular ego". In addition, Freud posits a primary hatred directed at whatever appears initially as an 'outside' to the subject: this, indeed, is "the ego's original reaction to objects in the external world" (p. 252).

Hatred is thus certainly a complicating factor in the mourning process, and it has at least three sources: particular experiences concerning the relation to the lost object, constitutional factors and the primary hatred of whatever is constituted as outside. As Freud (1915) would put it in his paper 'Thoughts on Time of War and Death', our loved ones are "inner possessions, components of our own ego" and also "purely strangers, even enemies" (Freud, 1915, p. 298). This combination of love and hate will lead quite logically to self-reproach following their death, predicated on the presence of unconscious death wishes. If we add to all this the sweep of the melancholic's narcissistic regression, do we have enough to account for the strange phenomenon of self-reproach in the melancholic subject?

Responses to Freud

Abraham and Klein certainly didn't think so, and in fact nor did any of the later analysts who tackled the problem in any sort of systematic way. The main thrust of the earlier revisions to Freud's paper was to weaken the distinction between mourning and melancholia that had appeared pivotal to Freud's argument. To start with, it was argued that ambivalence to the object – and hence reproach directed to it – was a feature at play in mourning and was by no means restricted to melancholia or pathological mourning. And, similarly, that introjection of the object was present in all forms of mourning. As we will see, these revisions all lost sight of the place of Freud's theory of narcissism in his explanation of melancholia.

Abraham had been engaged in a dialogue with Freud about melancholia for some time prior to the publication of the 1915 text, and Freud credits him with his emphasis on oral processes during mourning (Abraham, 1911). Although he had published several articles dealing with these issues, it was his 'Short Study of the Development of the Libido' published in 1924 that contained his fullest elaboration of the problems linked to the loss of an object (Abraham, 1924). Reading this text, it is difficult to ignore the fact that rumours of Freud's imminent death had been circulating shortly before Abraham put pen to paper, and a strange mechanism emerges in the Berlin analyst's prose: he repeatedly makes such statements as "psychoanalysis has thrown no light on [mourning] in healthy people and in cases of transference neurosis", a claim which is astounding given the sophistication of Freud's 1917 paper (Abraham, 1924, p. 434). He then invariably follows such statements – and there are plenty of them – with an obsequious reference to Freud, a rhythm which bears uncanny testimony to the very phenomenon of ambivalence that he argues is so crucial to the mourning process.

This ambivalence is found by Abraham (1924) at the heart of all mourning processes, which in turn are all derivatives of melancholia, which he takes to be the archaic form of mourning. In its basic melancholic form, the subject's hatred of their object swamps their love, and loss is experienced as an anal process while introjection is an oral one (p. 444). Both of these developmental levels have subdivisions: to expel and destroy on one level for the anal process, and to retain and control on the other, and sucking and pleasure on one level for the oral process with biting and destruction on the other. The object, he argues, is expelled like excrement, and then devoured. The subject's thirst for vengeance now finds satisfaction in tormenting the ego, a state which continues until sadistic tendencies have somehow been appeased and the love object removed from the danger of being destroyed. Thus, the mourning process ends when the subject has been liberated from the object, a process that is once again equated with shitting it out.

This gives the key to melancholia for Abraham. The melancholic subject tries to escape from his oral sadism and therefore turns his hatred against himself. The loss of the object evokes infantile disappointment from the mother while at the ambivalent stage of the developmental ladder. Thus, in Abraham's logic, self-reproach is ultimately a reproach to the mother. The feeling of hopelessness felt by the subject, in turn, is the result of the failure to achieve complete love or hatred of the object (Abraham, 1924, p. 469; Freud, 2002, pp. 303–305). But self-reproach may also have other sources: it may perpetuate the establishment of the lost object in the place of an ideal. A subject's complaints about himself may turn out to follow exactly the form of the mother's complaints about the subject. Or the reproach may echo that of one of the parents to the other. The attack on the object constituted by the reproach may have the form of an attack by a third party on the object: a subject's self-reproaches may echo those of the mother to the father, for example. All of these possibilities presuppose different patterns of identification and significantly broaden Freud's model of self-reproach.

Klein continued Abraham's research on melancholia, agreeing with him that melancholia and mourning were forms of the same structure. In a sense, the crucial hypothesis for both her and Abraham was that object relations develop in an ambivalent setting (Zetzel, 1953). Like Abraham, she disagreed with the supposedly Freudian idea that mourning, as opposed to melancholia, involved an unalloyed love. The loss of an object, she argued, will revive all the earlier losses that one has experienced and attributed to one's own destructive impulses. These circumstances will undermine any feelings of the secure possession of loved internal objects and will revive earlier anxieties about injured and damaged objects. Hence for Klein, "a successful reinstating of the external love object which is being mourned, and whose introjection is intensified through the process of mourning, implies that the loved internal objects are restored and regained" (Klein, 1952, p. 77).

Klein's theory of mourning entails that the straits of the depressive position will have to be run through once again with each significant loss later in life. The infantile prototype here is the state of mourning following the realisation in the depressive position that loved and hated objects are in fact aspects of the same object. This generates feelings of sadness and guilt, and subsequent attempts at reparation are understood as efforts to overcome mourning. As for self-reproach, this is taken to be the vehicle of both harm done to the object by hostile impulses and a more fundamental hatred of the id: in Klein's view, hatred of one's own hatred. This may be even more archaic than the previous form of hatred: the ego's very existence is threatened by the unleashing of hatred of the id, threatening the destruction of the ego's love objects (Klein, 1935, p. 270).

Each loss thus has a series of pernicious effects: good objects are threatened, and the subject is left at the mercy of a battery of bad objects. Hence the activation of the processes involved in the subject's passage through the depressive position, and, in particular, the ubiquitous phenomena of splitting observable after a loss. If early struggles around the loss of the mother had not been dealt with, depressive illness is more likely to ensue. Klein thus gives an answer to Freud's question about the pain involved in the mourning process. It involves, after all, a rebuilding of the internal world which is perceived as being in danger of collapsing (Klein, 1940, p. 354).

Although Klein and her students went on to elaborate and illustrate these ideas (Segal, 1952; Rosenfeld, 1959; Wisdom, 1962), psychoanalytic work on the themes set out in Freud's initial paper began to wane outside the Kleinian tradition. The term 'melancholia' more or less disappeared, to be replaced by that of 'depression' and its derivatives (Radden, 2000; Healy, 1997). Despite its abundance, the literature on depressive states, for the most part, lost sight of the issues that had been central to Freud's investigation. As for mourning, it received little attention outside the current of attachment theory established by John Bowlby (Bowlby, 1960, 1961, 1963). Bowlby's ideas can hardly be called psychoanalytic, and, from the early 1960s, he pursued a research programme that was explicitly based on a rejection of Freudian principles (A. Freud, 1960; Spitz, 1960). His attempts to theorise the mourning process dispense with the Freudian idea of identification with the lost object, and Bowlby seeks an adaptive explanation for such phenomena as self-reproach which underplays the role of sexuality and violence. In his view, reproach functions as a way to admonish the lost object to prevent it from disappearing again (Bowlby, 1961). Both reproach and self-reproach are described as preparations for an expected reunion or to undo loss.

Before turning to Lacan's contributions to these debates, what can we conclude from the post-Freudian revisions we have discussed? All the analytic commentators emphasise the presence of hatred and reproach to the object throughout the spectrum of mourning processes. They all seem to take for granted the fact that identification with the lost object is ubiquitous in both mourning and melancholia. Curiously, the view that mourning involves such identifications is often referred to Freud's 1915 paper, when he in fact says no such thing there. This is surprising in itself, given the mass of anthropological material on mourning rites that Freud was certainly familiar with. Homeopathy with the dead is perhaps the most common feature to be discerned by these studies, ranging from an adoption of the clothing of the deceased to an immersion in the dirt that the body would be buried in and, in general, some form of social seclusion for the bereaved. The pollution and withdrawal from society of the deceased's relatives is usually understood as a participation in their state (Seaford, 1994).

It is significant, then, to find that Freud (1923) would generalise his model of melancholic identification in 'The Ego and the Id', published some six years after 'Mourning and Melancholia' (p. 28). Such identifications are now seen as constitutive of the ego which is formed from abandoned object cathexes, but there is still no manifest reference to mourning here. How such identifications would differ from those involved in the process of mourning was not subsequently elaborated by Freud, and the main post-Freudian contributions to this problem tend to be isolated: perhaps the best examples are Edith Jacobson's (1954a & 1954b) superb papers from the 1950s exploring psychotic identifications and depression, and Vamik Volkan's (1981) insightful work on grief and mourning.

A further characteristic of the post-Freudian work on mourning and melancholia is the neglect of Freud's emphasis on the register of narcissism. Rosenfeld (1959) attempted to demonstrate, rather unconvincingly, that Klein's account of melancholia subsumes the Freudian theory of narcissism. The particularity of Klein's model here is that she takes the theory of mourning as in a very basic sense identical to the theory of the constitution of the subject. But where she claims that object loss leads to loss of one's inner objects, a Freudian perspective might suggest that these objects are the self, if we understand the latter term as designating a set of narcissistic identifications. Similar confusions pervade Jacobson's work, where the theory of narcissism is reformulated in terms of the dynamics between so-called self and object representations.

Likewise neglected are the effects of the social erosion of the rites of mourning, and, in general, a consideration of the dialectical relations between mourner and lost object; and, for that matter, the other significant players in the subject's constellation. Klein's work, however, stands out in its sensitivity to the phenomena after bereavement: the often-rigid splitting into good and bad polarities, the use of manic defences, and the ubiquitous dreams of damaging and repairing a body are all remarkably clear in such cases. It is quite tempting to imagine that Klein was inspired, certainly in her work of the 1930s, by her work with such patients.

Lacanian perspectives

As we noted at the start of our discussion, there are few references to mourning and melancholia in Lacan's published work. Mourning is discussed in some detail in the seminar 'Desire and Its Interpretation' (Lacan, 1958–1959), mentioned briefly in the 'Ethics' seminar, then slightly more extensively in the seminar on 'Transference', before largely disappearing from sight in the seminar transcripts (Lacan, 1992, pp. 354–6; 1991, pp. 439, 458–460). There are a handful of well-known remarks in the later written work: the references to the mourning at the end of the analysis and the "moral fault" of sadness and depression in '*Television*' (Lacan, 1974, p. 39). As for melancholia, there are some comments in the seminar on 'Dread' (Lacan, 2014) as well as in the other seminars we have listed.

As one might expect, the case has been made that, in fact, there are more numerous references to mourning and melancholia in Lacan's work, and that it is just a case of knowing how to read him properly. Hence the frequent appeal, for example, to passages in 'Function and Field of Speech and Language' which are assumed to be pertinent here (Lacan, 1966, p. 319; Laurent, 1988). Although the diagnosis of melancholia is often employed in case literature, we are told little about its metapsychology. The heroic exception here is the work of Christian Vereecken (1986 & 1993–1994), who has written extensively on melancholia over the last 20 years. More recently, there have been important studies by Geneviève Morel and her colleagues (2002), and by Frédéric Pellion (Morel, 2002; Pellion,

2000; Delacroix & Rein, 2001, bibliography). As for mourning, just as Freud's speculations were to be more or less unelaborated by future analysts, so Lacanian literature has been very reserved on the issue (Menard, 1982; Turnheim, 1997). Jean Allouch's (1995) remarkable book-length study on mourning is the exception here.

How is the question of mourning posed in Lacan's work? In the seminar 'Desire and Its Interpretation', it is through a reading of 'Hamlet' that a number of hypotheses are elaborated upon. Lacan sees the play as a study of man's relationship to desire. Since he takes desire to be supported by phantasy, it is Hamlet's relation to his phantasy object that becomes crucial to his perspectives on the play. Two problems confront the Prince, problems which have all their relevance for a study of mourning and bereavement today. First of all, the question of the father's knowledge: he knows too much, not simply in the sense of knowing the cause of his own death, but through the fact that he had not been able to prepare for his last rites, having been "interrupted, taken by surprise" so that "the possibility of response, of retribution, is sealed off forever" (Lacan, 1959–1960, 9 April 1959). Secondly, Hamlet has a mother who is unable to mourn: no sooner has her husband been killed than she opens her arms to another man. No mourning period is observed, no subjective loss is symbolised. When Hamlet confronts Gertrude, after contesting her position, he swiftly seems to give in, telling her that she can more or less do as she pleases. This indicates, for Lacan, a fall of desire for Hamlet: he is crushed by his mother's desire and is hence unable to situate properly his relation to his desire. In terms of the graph, $ \lozenge $ a has colonised S[]a.

Before examining Lacan's developments from these starting points, we can note how close they are to contemporary problems associated with loss. In his pioneering study on death, grief and mourning, Geoffrey Gorer (1965) drew attention to the fact that it had become commonplace to hide a patient's fatal diagnosis from them. Where Aries (1974) found a preparedness for death in earlier cultural testimonies, both he and Gorer see the contemporary problem as precisely this relation of death to knowledge. What questions, after all, are raised by the awareness of the impending death of one's own when this awareness is not shared? Likewise, the problem of how a parent has symbolised a loss is crucial for the mourning process: as we see again and again clinically, when a loss is not symbolised in family history, it so often returns to haunt the next generation. Contemporary culture inflects this problem in its own way: where children were once gathered around a deathbed, today we hear increasingly of their exclusion. Aries (1974) notes that until the eighteenth century, no portrayal of a deathbed scene failed to include children (p. 12). And where a parent decides it's for the good of the child to keep them away from a funeral, don't we hear about it decades later with a sense of disappointment or resentment, indicative that desire is at play?

Given the two problems which Lacan sees as establishing the framework of Hamlet's dilemma, how is the Prince able to re-find the place of his desire? Lacan's reading focuses on Hamlet's relationship with Ophelia: first rejected and humiliated, then valued and mourned. He sees Hamlet's relation to Ophelia as presenting a sort of model of the subject's relation to the object of desire. The rejection of Ophelia is interpreted as blocking the functioning of the imaginary structure of the phantasy: the debased image of the carnal woman that emerges from the scene with Gertrude intrudes to contaminate the place of Ophelia in Hamlet's desire. It is only after the scene in the cemetery that Hamlet can regain access to his desire when he is confronted with the image of the grieving Laertes. Laertes mourns where Hamlet has not, and it is through the homology of levels of the graph (d → ($ ◇ a)) and (m → i(a)) that Hamlet can assume his desire (Lacan, 1966, p. 816). The counterpart offers the image of the little other in relation to the object, and it is thus through the imaginary that Hamlet can move towards a position of mourning. Or, as Lacan (1959–1960) calls it, a "constitution of the object", made possible by an engagement with its inherent impossibility (22 April 1959).

What sort of impossibility is involved here? On an immediate level, it is the real loss of Ophelia that elevates her into an impossible object. The place of this object is constructed through the castration complex. The subject is deprived of part of his being, the signifier of which is the phallus: the object can then come into the place of what the subject is symbolically deprived of. This means that Ophelia can only take on her value given what Lacan calls "a mourning of the phallus". Hamlet's earlier rejection of Ophelia is interpreted as a rejection of the phallus, and this rejection has to move to the level of sacrifice in order to allow the reintegration of the object. This mourning of the phallus is how Lacan (1959–1960) characterises the *Untergang* of the Oedipus complex (29 April 1959).

Lacan's commentary not only opens up a number of new perspectives on the mourning process but also resonates in a particular way with Kleinian theory. As Allouch points out, Lacan's idea that mourning is only possible given the "constitution" of the object echoes Klein's well-known formula that "Not until the object is loved as a whole can its loss be felt as a whole" (Allouch, 1995, p. 52; Klein, 1935, p. 264). Although an appeal to wholeness is hardly a feature of Lacan's approach, both perspectives share the idea that, for mourning to operate, the object – and the object's place – has to be built up, and that this construction is never a given. Similarly, the reference to sacrifice allows us to situate the many burial rites that involve abandonment by the bereaved of a part of him- or herself, be it in the form of a lock of hair or some other object, that is thrown into the grave or tomb: the mourner's hair, unlike the mourner, will stay with the dead. Presumably, the characteristic of some cases is that the bereaved will identify with this jettisoned object so that the sacrifice involves not a part of the subject, but the subject as such.

Lacan's discussion also raises the question of the place of someone else's mourning for the subject. It is through the spectacle of Laertes' mourning, after all, that Hamlet can access his own. This dialogue of mourning is a motif we find described repeatedly in literature and poetry. We could cite, for example, the scene in the 'Illiad' following the death of Patroklos, where the women lament his passing openly while, at the same time, "each one for her own sorrows", and the men "each one remembering what he had left at home" (Illiad 19: 302). The public mourning ritual for the dead warrior serves to polarise the memories of earlier losses for those present. Indeed, it has been argued that the lamentation for long-dead heroes that had such a precise place in Hellenistic culture had the function of providing a space for the bewailing of individual, private losses (Seaford, 1994).

This dialogue of mourning finds an echo in Klein's work. In her 1940 paper on mourning and its relations to manic-depressive states, she makes a few rather tantalising remarks about the work of mourning sometimes being precipitated if one's internal objects are mourning with one (Klein, 1940, pp. 359–362). This idea of a relation between mournings, or a 'borrowed mourning', is developed implicitly by Hanna Segal (1952) in a classic article on aesthetics. Segal elaborates on Kleinian concepts to provide a framework to understand the aesthetic experience. After a discussion of the concept of sublimation, she makes a very simple but also barely noticed point about the experience of works of art: although at some level we might believe that we 'identify' with the protagonists, there is also a process of identification with the creator, in the sense of someone who could make something out of an inferred experience of loss. As Segal (1952) puts it, they have created something "out of chaos and destruction" (p. 199).

This may seem like a trivial point, and we might certainly disagree with Segal's explanations, but it indicates the significance of exposure to the manifest mourning process of someone else. Segal goes on to argue that it is through "identifying with the artist" that successful mourning can be achieved, implying a rather transitory experience of catharsis rather than the drawn-out work of mourning described by Freud. However, if we follow her Kleinian approach and see all creative works as being products of the same mechanisms, the place of art in culture takes on a new sense: a set of instruments to help us to mourn. This was already a motif in Plato's 'Republic' where we can read how "poets gratify and indulge the natural desire to weep and lament to our heart's content, which in our private misfortune we forcibly restrain" (Republic 605c–606b; Seaford, 1994, p. 140).

The notion of a dialogue of mournings that we can extract from Lacan and Klein is not intended to suggest that witnessing someone else's mourning will necessarily engender mourning in the subject; it is even less to suggest that, if mourning does get underway, it will be extensive, sustained or successful. The other's mourning can act as an imaginary route for the subject, but not more than that. This process can shed light on other phenomena to the extent that it alerts us to the active effects of comparison. Finding an imaginary representation that echoes our own situation can, as we have seen, initiate a mourning process, but what about instances where the very possibility of comparison seems to be ruled out?

The most evident – and perhaps the only – example of such a barrier in our culture is the Holocaust. When Sylvia Plath dared to use images of the Holocaust in her poem 'Daddy' to situate personal, autobiographical threads, the response was outrage and anger (Malcom, 1993, pp. 64–65). If we take seriously the argument about the resonance between mournings, this produces a number of problems: in particular, the seal of the prohibition on the comparison that marks representations of the Holocaust disallows the pattern of mourning we have discussed to take place. On a clinical level, we could find examples of the unavailability of comparisons in the very simple notion of the absence of symbolisation of some loss in a family. As we have seen, Hamlet didn't find it in Gertrude and had to wait until the encounter with the grieving Laertes.

This can tell us something about both mourning and memory. Mark Roseman's (2000) book, 'The Past in Hiding', tells the story of Marianne Ellenbogen, a young Jewish woman who survived underground in Nazi Germany. Roseman's narrative does not rely simply on the interviews he had with Marianne but also draws on her contemporary diaries, together with information gathered from several other sources. The book is rare in its bold handling of a difficult subject: what interests Roseman is less to paint a picture of heroism and valour than to examine the tensions between fiction and non-fiction in Marianne's narrative. Her diaries from the war often tell a very different story from her later reconstructions, just as both of these sources sometimes conflict with external accounts (Roseman, 1999).

As Roseman scrutinised the material, a certain pattern became clear. Where moments of separation were so traumatic as to be unbearable for the subject, they would be rewritten using the memories of other people. How should this strange phenomenon be understood? It is less a question of so-called false memory syndrome than that of the principle of borrowed mourning: the stories that Marianne would substitute for the unspeakable points in her narrative concerned someone else grieving a loss, together with little details about the circumstances of that loss. Although, as Roseman shows, these losses were not her own, can't we see them as instruments that allowed her to mourn? This phenomenon might remind us of the process of hysterical identification, where a common element is found due to a shared experience of lack. The subject puts themself in the place of someone else because of the imputation of lack to that person, as we see in the famous examples discussed by Freud (1899, pp. 149–151).

But is the process we have been discussing really so similar to hysterical identification? This is far from certain and takes us back to the question we posed earlier about the curious paucity of psychoanalytic literature on mourning. The contrast between fiction and poetry seems remarkable, and indeed, the majority of British first novels today are about death. Since psychoanalysts experience losses, just like everyone else, why should they shy away from writing about them? There are of course notable exceptions here, and we could mention the many papers on mourning written by George Pollock (1961), which began, as he says, after the death of his mother. But these remain the exception rather than the rule. Why should analysts tread warily on the borders of what writers of fiction seem to embrace so eagerly?

Aside from the good reasons for an aversion to broadcasting the details of one's private life, perhaps we can find a more structural explanation here, even a clue as to some of the mechanisms that mourning involves. We could start by making a clinical observation: it seems curious that artists often say so little about their work in analysis. They can talk about just about everything else, their rivals, their dealers, their partners and so forth, but not about what they are actually doing. It seems possible that one reason for this might be that the processes which result in the creation of works are separate from those predicated on repression. Might it be the case, then, that the avoidance of the theme of mourning implies that we aren't dealing with repression here but with other mechanisms, and that hence to circumscribe it we have to use fictional prose or other means of creative expression?

There is perhaps a hint of this in Lacan's (1959–1960) discussion of mourning. He has very little to say here about repression, and, surprisingly, compares mourning – in an inverted way – with the mechanism constitutive of psychotic structure: foreclosure (22 April 1959). In a psychosis, we see the return in the Real of elements foreclosed from the symbolic. In mourning, Lacan argues, we see the opposite: a real loss is treated with a mobilisation of the totality of the symbolic. Here again, we find an echo of Klein, who stressed how mourning involved the mobilisation of the totality of the internal world of the subject, not just the representations of the lost object but the whole set of representations of all objects. Lacan's immediate reference here is to burial rites, a set of purely formal practices in which the mourner participates. The formal nature of such rites has indeed generated endless debates in anthropology around the question of whether emotions evinced on such occasions are 'genuine', and hence whether emotions give rise to rites or an effect of them (Metcalf & Huntington, 1991). Lacan's emphasis on the signifier allows us to avoid the pitfalls of these debates: if the symbolic is being mobilised as a totality, there will be an emphasis on precisely those structures that have the highest symbolic density, distanced from the field of imaginary meanings.

Given this comparison, the odd imaginary phenomena found in mourning, such as quasi-hallucinatory experiences, become less surprising: if the symbolic is replying as such to a hole in the real, imaginary elements will be mobilised, just as they are in the inverted process in psychosis. Lacan's idea is that although the symbolic is mobilised, signifying elements are inadequate to cope with the hole opened up by a loss. Hence, the folkloric and phantasmagorical battery of ghosts and ghouls, polarised when mourning rites have been abandoned or curtailed. Mourning rites function as a mediation of the gap opened up by a loss and involve the establishment of a correspondence between this gap and the symbolic lack. The phallus is the crucial signifier here, and it will be projected into the hole opened up by the loss, but since the phallus as a signifier cannot be articulated as such, the many disturbing images so often observed in the mourning process will assail the mourner at this point of symbolic lack (Lacan, 1959–1960, 29 April 1959).

As Lacan elaborated his theory of the object as real in the early 1960s, he returns to the theme of mourning in the seminar on anguish (Lacan, 2014). Hamlet, he reminds us, shows what mourning is all about – that is, the effort to restore the link to the lost object. We can note here a bizarre convergence of Lacan with Bowlby: both question the Freudian view that the detailed work of mourning is about separating. But where Bowlby sees it as the attempt to reunite with the lost object, Lacan sees it as an attempt to restore the place of the object, which supposes the subject's abandoning of a part of himself. We see the radical nature of Lacan's views on mourning: it is not about giving up an object but about restoring one's links to an object as lost, as impossible. The key here is to distinguish the object from the imaginary envelope that cloaks it.

If the links to the object are restored, and the place of the imaginary envelope discerned from this, it may become possible for another $i(a)$ to take its place. The problem for the mourner, Lacan argues, is that of maintaining links to $i(a)$, through which love is narcissistically structured. Mourning and melancholia are now distinguished in terms of these variables: a must be separated from $i(a)$, and it is in an attempt to reach himself as a that the melancholic may pass to the act in the suicidal scenarios that involve exiting from the 'stage' (Lacan, 2014, sessions of 16 January 1963 and 3 July 1963). If, in mourning, it is a question of the constitution of the object, and hence of a re-establishment of the subject's relation to the object in phantasy, in melancholia, such a "constitution" is not possible: instead, the subject gravitates towards the place of a separated from the signifying framework or, as Lacan puts it, "the stage of the world".

A clinical example can illustrate the functioning of these concepts. The patient had lost his wife a year previously and had been in a state of inertia since her death, unable to work or carry out his daily activities, haunted by images and memories of her, searching the streets for her image, and unable to maintain links with his friends and family. The sequence we can examine here took place over a six-month period, at the end of which he was able to overcome the severity of his inertial state, resume activities and think anew about the possibilities of living. I have chosen to focus on a series of dreams as they seem indicative of what allowed the mourning process to take place and signalled for this patient the presence of change.

Dream 1: X is furious with his wife, and they have a huge fight. He reproaches her for having failed to disclose certain information to him. Another woman then enters the scene, who has exaggerated traits of his wife. He leaves with her, and as they move through a party, he finds himself behaving with her the way his wife would behave in public with him. On waking, X contemplates for a moment the visual image of the second woman and suddenly realises that this is, in fact, the image of his wife.

Dream 2: X is in the house he had lived in with his wife. He wants a cup of tea, but there is no milk. He asks various characters who seem to be hanging around and is told that there is not enough milk left. He then goes into each room of the house, expecting to find someone there but there is no one. Finally, in the last room, X sees a multitude of belongings set out either in preparation for a trip or indicating the return from a trip. He expects to see his wife, but there's no one there.

Dream 3: X is in a shop. He drops some milk and hopes that the cashier will give him another carton for free. She doesn't. He then brings out all his change, but she still refuses. His wife appears and they cling to each other in a very physical, erotic way.

Dream 4: X is with his wife. She says, 'It's one-way traffic'. X tries to understand what this means. Is it one-way traffic for him, or his wife? He tries to understand but is unable to. Throughout the dream, X has the profound sensation of not knowing his wife. He then finds himself in a room filled with suitcases. He says either 'Been somewhere?' or 'Going somewhere?' but cannot remember which.

Dream 5: X is with his wife and again has the sensation of her strangeness. She seems alien, completely opaque. Then she takes hold of him and says, 'Don't ever leave me'. He says, 'I won't', but isn't actually too sure.

Dream 6: X feels out of place. Then there is simply an image of a piece of white fabric with a small excremental stain on it.

One could certainly approach these dreams from the usual perspectives of popular psychology: the denial of death, the rage, the journey, the parting, etc. But they reveal far more of the processes that allow mourning to take place. Note first of all, in Dream 1, that the reproach to the wife in fact echoed the subject's reproach to his mother at a particular moment in his childhood, a reproach that had not been conscious to X until he was associating to the dream. The doubling of women and X's identificatory behaviour index the imaginary register, and, as we'll see, the parameter of narcissism. Dream 2 also evokes X's relation to his mother, who had "run out of milk" after a brief period of breastfeeding X. The third dream continues this refinement of the separation of the field of narcissism and the object: when X is confronted with a woman who refuses to give him anything, the image of his wife appears, and bodily enjoyment responds to the point of frustration. In terms of the analytic work during this time, it was a question of the object situated in his wife and the relations of this to the representations of his mother.

Dreams 4 and 5 are in a way paradigmatic of the mourning process, in demonstrating the separation of the image and the real register beyond it. Both of them confront X with the intense sensation of something unknowable about his wife. The question about the meaning of the one-way traffic evoked for X both the one-way journey of his wife and the fact that he too would be taking a one-way journey at some point in the future. His incomprehension can be taken as a sign of the real, where death presents itself as an opaque riddle to which the subject – and indeed the signifier – has no answer. The questions about the meaning of the baggage also reminded X of an important time in his childhood when his mother had left on a trip without any prior warning. These themes are played out again in the fifth dream around the phrase: 'Don't ever leave me', which X would ascribe to himself, addressed both to his mother and his wife.

Before commenting on the apparently incongruous sixth dream, we should say something about X's experience since (roughly) the time of Dream 4. These months had been characterised by an overcoming of inertia and an almost manic enjoyment taken in certain jokes, wordplays and anecdotes that he would return to frequently. After Dream 6, X realised that all the jokes, wordplays, and anecdotes actually shared a common theme: a scatological reference to the anal child. The shift in the dream from the subject not having a place to his total eclipse in the image of the excrementally marked fabric gave the equivalence of the subject to the object. At this moment, X remembered a detail from the period during which he had first met his wife. Before the dinner at which he had been introduced to her, he had heard a story about a holiday scene in which she had apparently relieved herself in an uninhibited display. In the following weeks, X would remember his efforts to hide his excretory activities as a child from everyone but his mother.

X's dreams were not interpreted by the analyst. Instead, they were interpreted by X himself, and in a certain sense, like many of the dreams we find punctuating the mourning process, they were interpretations in themselves. Although we might choose to find in them the anal dynamics that so interested Abraham, it seems to me that they bring out the split between the field of narcissistic identification and the object emphasised by Lacan. In the dream series, we see a separation of the image of the wife from the oral and anal object, and in the associations, the thread that made this woman take the place in his phantasy that she held for so long, a thread that had one foot in the field of narcissism. In Dream 6, we see how the lack of a signifier responds to the point of real loss. At the end of the sequence, in X's new interest in life, we see, broadly speaking, the reintegration of the object in its narcissistic framework.

These dreams also illustrate the dialectic of desires that Lacan put at the heart of the mourning process. The opacity of the woman and her enigmatic pronouncement index the dimension of the desire of the Other, and the object emerges as a response. The question here concerns, as Lacan put it, to what extent the subject was a lack for the Other, that is, what place they had in their desire. Although the subject's 'Don't ever leave me' is ascribed to the wife, her ineffable and opaque presence in the previous dreams was experienced as a fundamental non-recognition, indicating that her desire was aimed ultimately beyond him. When Lacan observed that we can only mourn someone of whom we can say 'I was their lack', it precisely implies this question of what we were for the Other (Lacan, 2014, session of 30 January 1963). In this sense, part of the work of mourning involves mourning the imaginary object that we were for the Other. And isn't hatred one of the consequences of not being able to say, 'I was their lack'? Exactly what blocks the mourning process, according to Freud.

Does mourning end?

X was able to overcome his inertia, and, after a certain time, to reacquire a taste for life and his interest in the opposite sex. But should we speak here of a completed mourning? Analytic writers have been divided on this issue: "Mourning is for life" said Margaret Little, and although a clinician with the acumen of Helene Deutsch could speak of a necessity to mourn, she was later sceptical about any 'completion' of 'internal processes' (Little, 1986, p. 301; Deutsch, 1937, pp.

20–21; Deutsch, 1966). Freud, likewise, took care to point out how a loss could never be entirely compensated for. In a 1929 letter to Binswanger, he wrote: "We will never find a substitute [after a loss]. No matter what may fill the gap, even if it be filled completely, it nevertheless remains something else. And actually, this is how it should be, it is the only way of perpetuating that love which we do not want to relinquish" (Freud, 2001).

This statement might be compared with Freud's remark in the 1908 paper on 'Creative Writers', where he says that "We can never give anything up: we only exchange one thing for another" (Freud, 1908, p. 145). It seemed to analysts like Pollock that where we assume a mourning process to have been run through, residual phenomena remained which indicated that this was far from the case. The most conspicuous of these were the so-called 'anniversary' reactions, where the subject would develop symptoms on reaching the age of the deceased, or that of a third party linked to the deceased. Pollock (1970) observed that in cases where the father's death occurred before that of the mother, anniversary symptoms often emerged upon reaching the age of the mother at the time of the father's death.

Pollock saw one aim of the analytic approach as allowing memories to take the place of anniversary reactions, but he also felt that certain losses could never be adequately mourned: for example, that of a mother for a dead child. This raises several questions, and the documented prevalence of anniversary symptoms suggests that, in fact, most bereaved people have not 'got over' their loss. Presumably, we should not shy away from this kind of generalisation, but equally, we should not shy away from the question of whether the idea of 'getting over' a loss has any real meaning. One way of exploring this question is through the idea of the preconditions for mourning (Wolfenstein, 1966). Is mourning possible, for example, without speech? Does it require the prior passage through the depressive position, the dissolution of the Oedipus complex, the trial of adolescence or the many other phases, stages and complexes that analysts have vaunted?

For Freud and Abraham, one of the major preconditions for mourning involved the analysis of ambivalence surrounding the deceased. For Klein, a more or less positive introjection (or re-introjection) of the lost object should occur together with that of the archaic 'good' object. For Jacobson, the mourner must identify with the so-called 'positive' aspects of the lost object. The mourner will experience guilt and self-reproach, but without the sort of globalising, regressive identification characteristic of melancholia. Different, less enveloping identifications will indicate the movement through the mourning process. This might seem at odds with Freud's 1915 thesis, where he states that the work of mourning must declare the object to be dead. But in fact, this is not contradictory with the presence of certain identificatory processes: in 'The Ego and the Id', after all, he tells us that such identifications are constitutive of the ego as such, and that giving up an object perhaps always involves some form of identification.

Declaring the object to be dead, however, is by no means a simple process. And, in fact, it might imply nothing less than killing the dead. In a letter to Jones, Freud notes that the work of mourning involves "bringing the recognition of the reality principle to every point of the libido ... one then has the choice of dying oneself or of acknowledging the death of the loved one, which again comes very close to your expression that one kills this person" (Freud, in Paskauskas, 1993, pp. 652–653). It has been observed that dreams involving a dreamer's murderous attack on the deceased sometimes indicate a rather positive prognosis (Volkan, 1981, p. 64). And real death is hardly the same thing as a proper, symbolic death, as the many rites and superstitions surrounding the dead show so clearly. We talk in whispers around a dead person and arrange the paraphernalia of burial so as to prevent the return of the deceased. Anthropologists have repeatedly pointed out how burial rites aim to keep the dead at bay: heavy coffins, tokens and sacrifices all arguably have this palliative and protective function. The animism ascribed to the dead is yet one more sign that we are never quite sure that they aren't about to come back.

Part of the originality of Lacan's approach was in linking this Freudian question of declaring the object dead with the theme of narcissistic investment. Freud argued that the mourner had a choice: either to follow the dead or to follow the narcissistic investments of living. But Lacan went a step further by associating this choice with that of the subject at the time of the dissolution of the Oedipus complex. The subject must choose between the narcissistic investment of the penis and the incestuous demands aimed at the mother. Although he reformulates the Freudian choice in terms of the imaginary and symbolic sides to the phallus, he is situating the problem of mourning within the history of the subject's relation to castration. And, if the sacrifice of the phallus constitutive of the dissolution of the Oedipus complex establishes chains of representations forbidden to the subject, mourning emerges as the precondition of desire as such.

The choice described by Freud, and reformulated by Lacan, between dying oneself or declaring the object dead is thus a crucial variable in the mourning process. We will see in the next section how the first option is often chosen in melancholia, but with the second, we have to ask how such a declaration can take place. In Lacanian terms, it involves the sacrifice of the phallus. And this will have a number of consequences, one of which concerns the nature of the subject's debt. Commentators have often noted how although a bereaved person seems to be getting on with the mourning process, the possibility of new attachments remains blocked. Mourning has its time, but what we see so frequently is the question of loyalty to the dead which conflicts with ties to the living. When a symbolic debt remains confused with an imaginary one, the framework of pathological mourning may be established. This was perhaps exactly the problem faced by the Ratman. And hence, at times, the clinical efficacity of an emphatic acknowledgement of the symbolic side to a subject's debt.

Freud's account of the process of mourning involves, as we've seen, the idea of exhaustion of representations. As the representations of the lost object are hypercathected and the memories and hopes linked to it are met by the judgement that the object no longer exists, so the work of mourning will gradually exhaust itself. But how might such a process be distinguished from one in which the subject remains haunted by representations? What, after all, is to stop the piecemeal process described by Freud from continuing forever? At what point does the cycle exhaust itself, if at all? Lacan's formulation suggests that in addition to this aspect of the work of mourning, the subject's phallic sacrifice must be reactualised. Allouch (1995) has indeed given such a central place to this notion that he encourages us to see mourning not as a 'work' but rather as an 'act'. What else might one infer here in terms of the dynamic of representations?

One way of formulating these themes might be to pursue the distinction made by the Russian Formalists and adopted by Lacan, between a representation and a representation of a representation. If we assume that each representation linked to the lost object is heavily cathected, we might expect a libidinal shift to occur if it becomes possible to make these representations into a set, which is then represented as such. As Franz Kaltenbeck (2002) points out, if representations are not gathered up into a set, the subject remains haunted by them. This was one of the effects of the establishment of the paternal metaphor for Lacan, where the sliding of meanings is rendered finite by the phallic signification. One indication of this process is the emphasis on the representation as such, its nature as a representation, and this is made possible by the addition of a border or a frame.

A border, in the form of a frame, a window or an arch, for example, allows what is seen to be situated as a representation. And to perceive some representation as a representation, in other words, as a sign system, it is necessary to designate its borders. Indeed, in many languages, the word for 'limit' is etymologically related to that for 'represent' (Uspensky, 1973, p. 140). We might note the fact here that those investigating mourning have been struck by the ubiquity, at a certain moment in the process, of dreams featuring frames (Volkan, 1981, p. 163). And, as is well known, Lacan (2014) would also appeal to the theory of frames and windows to elaborate his theory of the phantasy, especially in the context of a discussion of mourning and melancholia (see session of 16 January 1963).

Similarly, if we follow Lacan's argument contrasting mourning and foreclosure, the mobilisation of the symbolic in response to the hole in the real suggests another comparison. The hole in the Real of mourning and the hole in the symbolic of psychosis both entail consequences at the level of the imaginary, and this imbrication of registers calls to mind some of Lacan's remarks about phobia. Phobia, for the Lacan of 1956, involves the work of reshuffling imaginary elements, to situate a new symbolic configuration that responds to the emergence of the real (Lacan, 1994, p. 343). The interest of this comparison in terms of mourning is that the theory of registers implies that just as in a phobia we will see an accentuation of the properties of a representation as a representation (Little Hans' crumpled giraffe) due to the reshuffling process, so we will see in mourning an emphasis or enhancement of the semiotic qualities of a representation. This signals a shift from a representation of a so-called reality (that of the loved object) to a representation of a representation of this reality.

These indications are compatible with the theory of mourning that Lacan elaborated in the seminar on 'Desire and its Interpretation' if we correlate the constitution of the object with set-theoretical changes in the signifier. Lacan would later introduce a theory of separation, taking the term not from the tradition of attachment theory but rather from medieval philosophy, to formulate the subject's separation from the signifying chain (Lacan, 2014, see session of 30 January 1963; Owens, 1972; Schmidt, 1960). The implication is that without the constitution of the object necessary for separation, the subject remains tied to the signifying chain. And isn't this a definition in itself of a failure of mourning? It's not that one signifier represents the subject for another signifier, but that all signifiers represent the subject. Whereas for the mourner, one cracked paving stone is the conduit to a host of acute memories and affects, without separation everything becomes a cracked paving stone.

To make one further point about the preconditions of mourning, we should return to the theme of rites that so interested Lacan. In a sense, the preconditions of mourning are the rites of mourning. Gorer and other scholars not only recorded the progressive disappearance of such rites but lamented them. For Gorer, where the great taboo of Victorian culture was sex, today it is death. We might object that today we are continually assailed by images of violent death, in the cinema, on television and in all of culture's media. But one could see, in turn, this ramification as a strict consequence of the disappearance of rites. Without the symbolic support of mourning rites, images of death simply proliferate. And this absence of ritual has effects in the flesh: researchers have observed how physical symptoms in the bereaved are much more frequent in those geographical regions where the ritual is least present (Gorer, 1965, p. 49). At the end of his survey, Gorer encouraged the invention of new, secular mourning rituals. Since there is little evidence that anything comparable has taken place, it is up to each subject, perhaps, to invent their own. The space to do this is one of the offers of psychoanalysis.

The melancholic choice

Freud's paper contains a comment that seems to undermine his main argument. As he charts the differences between mourning and melancholia, he remarks that the litanies of the melancholic subject might in fact be similar to the detail work of the mourner and that the iterated reproaches might loosen the link to the lost object (Freud, 1917, p. 253, 257). "Each single struggle of ambivalence loosens the fixation of the libido to the object by disparaging it, denigrating it and even as it were killing it" (p. 257). These comments are surprising since it would seem that the whole binary structure of Freud's argument relies on the difference between the two structures and, furthermore, that the litanies of the melancholic take on their meaning, precisely due to a failure of the mourner's 'detail work', just as the reproaches of the melancholic would seem to be symptomatic of the object's inert presence in the ego rather than an attempt to shift it.

Freud's inclusion of these comments deserves to be taken seriously. Clinically, it is far from obvious that the melancholic plaint exhausts itself or loosens the link to the object, although both Klein and Abraham seem to have had some idea of progressive exhaustion in the melancholic subject. The stability of the plaint contrasts with the shifting detail work of the mourner. More generally, Freud's comments raise the question of the possible resolution of the sequences of both mourning and melancholia. To formulate this in melancholia, we need to return to the Freudian theory of representations and pinpoint one aspect of the melancholic relation to the signifier.

We often find in cases of melancholia a description of a split existence: on the one hand, a life lived with others in society and groups, and on the other the utter solitude of the subject. This should not be confused with the feeling of alienation often complained of by the neurotic. It may involve the idea that other beings are mere simulacra, unreal shadows, although once again this should be distinguished from the idea we find in paranoia that the simulacra are there for a reason. For the melancholic subject, there is often no reason, simply the testimony of an experience. Now, how might such phenomena be understood?

The standard Lacanian explanation is to appeal to the notion of topical regression to the mirror phase, an idea that Lacan (1966) develops in the 'Preliminary Question' (p. 568). Given the foreclosure of the Name of the Father and the opening up of a gulf in the imaginary, the subject is left with the mortal relation to the image and the aggressive erotised imaginary of the mirror phase. This topical regression is often evoked to situate the particular alienation of the melancholic, although, as Vereecken points out, Lacan uses it in fact to account for certain phenomena in paranoia. For Vereecken (1993–1994), the melancholic's difficulties here are at the level of secondary narcissism and do not involve a topical regression to the mirror phase (p. 89).

If we wish to inflect the more common view of a topical regression, another perspective might be introduced here. As we explore the childhood and upbringing of these subjects, we are often able to locate episodes quite early on in which the identity of someone close to the subject is doubted or appears as simulacra. As Lacanians, we tend to see these episodes as elementary phenomena and, as such, self-explanatory. But, in these clinical scenarios, we tend to be dealing with caregivers who are severely inconsistent, who change their aspect radically from one moment to the next in ways that an infant must find difficult to make sense of. Or, scenarios in which there is a sudden changing of hands, a movement from one caregiver to another at a particular point in the subject's history.

One solution, perhaps to these terrible circumstances would be to imagine that the caregiver is actually more than one person or an unreal one. Naturally, this reminds one of Klein's observations of splitting in infancy where, prior to the unification of the depressive position, the mother, and part objects, are seen as separate entities rather than aspects of one and the same entity. The psychotic phenomenon linked to simulacra seems to invite two different approaches: one structural, the other more linked to the history of the subject's object relations. These are not contradictory, since, for the assumption of doubling and simulacra to take place, we can posit the presence of foreclosure.

The split between the 'unreal' world and 'real' existence described by some melancholic subjects allows further comparisons between these two psychoanalytic approaches. As Lacanians, we would tend to understand reports of such experiences as a consequence of foreclosure: the 'real' world inhabited by such subjects involves such terrifying motifs as endless purgatory, minutes that last centuries, unutterable pain and angst, the call of the dead and so on. We would tend, perhaps, to simply class all these phenomena together as phi zero, without risking the kind of investigation that would differentiate the motifs in detail and explore their genesis. Perhaps the weight of Lacan's structural arguments against the content-based interpretations of Katan and Niederland regarding the Schreber case was rather discouraging (Lacan, 1966, pp. 542–543, 580).

And yet a Freudian argument can nuance our structural perspectives. The mourning subject, Freud (1917) says, when confronted with the question of whether it shall share the object's fate, "is persuaded by the sum of the narcissistic satisfactions it derives from being alive to sever its attachment to the object that has been abolished" (p. 255). If we assume that, in some cases, the subject in fact dies with their object, while avoiding suicide, one of the consequences is a split world. Dying with the object means that the object cannot be given up. Inhabiting the social world will contrast with the subject's participation in the world of the dead, an involvement that may only become manifest at rare moments. This dual participation is crucial from a clinical standpoint. Not to interpret it to the subject – since, after all, the subject knows it better than us – but rather to allow a sensitivity to the efforts to find a way of circumscribing this dual existence with the signifier. Not to emphasise one or the other, but rather to find signifiers to index the relation between them.

A melancholic subject is in two places at once, two entirely different spaces that cannot be superimposed. How can this impossible experience be communicated? In one case, where the subject decided to kill the analyst, although one could choose to appeal to all the motifs of oral sadism and hate made popular by Abraham and Klein, it became clear that his intention was simply to give the clinician an idea of the world he inhabited beyond that of social simulacra. This is ultimately a problem linked to language and the signifier, and we see the melancholic subject try repeatedly to find new ways to express the experience of impossibility. This is one reason for the loquaciousness of the melancholic that Freud noted with initial puzzlement. And perhaps this is why the theme of melancholy has historically always been linked to that of poetic creation.

This brings us to a sense of melancholic self-reproach quite distinct from those we have discussed previously. A melancholic subject can, in some cases, continue their litany of self-denigration, in the very precise sense of being not worthy of doing some duty which, as we explore it, is linked to a duty of speaking properly about the lost love object and their relation to it. This is absolutely not the problem of the neurotic subject. Neurotics are generally more concerned with problems of meaning and signification than with the basic problem of reference. A melancholic subject, however, can reproach himself endlessly for not being able to tell you with exactitude about something, not being able to reach something: the problem here is the basic impossibility of making words touch their referent. Hence the emergence, at times, of passages to the act which aim to do just that. Since words tend not to touch their referent, making them do so may involve violence – and this was interpreted by many post-Freudian authors exclusively as oral sadism and hate. To put it another way, the melancholic subject reproaches himself for failing to make the two worlds coincide, to generate an unbearable sense of impossibility that is distinct from the pain of mourning where the affect can be fractioned by the serial work of moving through representations of the object.

This variety of self-reproach is certainly not the only one to be found in melancholia, but we find it in enough cases to suggest that it warrants attention. One of the many merits of Pellion's recent study of melancholia is exactly this emphasis on what we could call the linguistic situation of the melancholic. A sensitivity to this relation to language can be significant for clarifying the place of passages to the act, which may on occasion be triggered when the clinician puts undue emphasis on one or the other of the melancholic's 'worlds'. Acting out is often distinguished from passages to the act in neurosis in terms of its demonstrative function: acting out is intended to convey some message to the Other, whereas passages to the act short circuit the dimension of the message. However, melancholic passages to the act sometimes precisely involve a demonstrative function, where an appeal is made to the Other as witness to an impossible situation. This differs from some passages to the act in paranoia where the capital issue for the subject is to obtain an admission from the Other.

We noted earlier on that the standard binary separating melancholia from paranoia derived from the efforts of late nineteenth-century psychiatry to generate symmetries between delusions of persecution and negation. A common perspective today involves a contrast between melancholic and paranoiac relations to the lack in the Other: for the paranoiac, it is interpreted as persecutory, as the site of *jouissance*, while for the melancholic it remains a hole, uninterpreted as such. However, there is an interest in nuancing the rather black-and-white terms of this binary. Certain cases of melancholia suggest that the relation to the Other is basically persecutory, but that this is kept at bay precisely through the melancholic introjection of the lost object. When what seems to be a melancholia shifts into a paranoia, the usual response is to assume that the case was simply a misdiagnosed paranoia, but what is of great interest here are those cases where, despite everything, no such shift occurs. The subject's attachment to a loss seems to have an ineradicable defensive function, an idea that perhaps echoes Klein's thesis that depressive states are structurally based on paranoid ones.

From a clinical angle, a melancholia can certainly improve. But this won't be due to its transformation into a mourning. Mourning, after all, involves the process of establishing the denial of a positive term. Melancholia, on the other hand, involves the affirmation of a negative term. As logic shows us, it is not possible to translate one into the other: predicate negation and term negation are fundamentally incompatible (Horn, 1989). In Freudian terms, with certain cases of melancholia, our aim might be less to try to access so-called thing representations than to allow the subject to find signifiers to index the impossibility of the passage from word to thing representations, from one representational system to the other. And isn't that one of the functions of poetry? As our lost colleague and friend Elizabeth Wright (1999) observed, melancholic subjects "require the poetic to deliver them" (p. 40).

References

Abraham, K. (1911). Notes on the psychoanalytical investigation and treatment of manic-depressive insanity and allied conditions. In *Selected Papers on Psychoanalysis* (pp. 137–156). London: Maresfield Reprints, 1979.

Abraham, K. (1924). A short study of the development of the libido viewed in the light of mental disorders. In *Selected Papers on Psychoanalysis* (pp. 418–501). London: Maresfield Reprints, 1979.

Allouch, J. (1995). *Erotique du deuil au temps de la mort seche*. Paris: EPEL.

Aries, P. (1974). *Western Attitudes Toward Death From the Middle Ages to the Present*. Baltimore: Johns Hopkins University Press.

Aries, P. (1977). *L'Homme devant la Mort*. Paris: Seuil.

Babb, L. (1951). *Elizabethan Malady: A Study of Melancholia in English Literature from 1580 to 1642*. East Lansing: Michigan State University Press.

Bowlby, J. (1960). Grief and mourning in infancy and early childhood. *Psychoanalytic Study of the Child*, 15, 9–52.

Bowlby, J. (1961). Processes of mourning. *International Journal of Psychoanalysis*, *42*, 317–340.

Bowlby, J. (1963). Pathological mourning and childhood mourning. *Journal of the American Psychoanalytic Association*, *11*, 500–541.

Capdevila L., & Voldman, D. (2002). *Nos Morts: Les societes occidentales face aux tues de la guerre*. Paris: Payot.

Delacroix, C., & Rein, G. (2001). Bibliographie sue melancolie et depression. *Figures de Psychanalyse*, *4*, 125–133.

Deutsch, H. (1937). Absence of grief. *Psychoanalytic Quaterly*, *6*, 12–23.

Deutsch, H. (1966). Posttraumatic amnesias and their adaptive function. In R. Loewenstein, L. Newman, & A. Solnit (Eds.), *Psychoanalysis: A General Psychology* (pp. 437–455). New York: International University Press.

Freud, A. (1960). Discussion of Dr. John Bowlby's paper. *Psychoanalytic Study of the Child*, *15*, 53–62.

Freud, S. (1899). The interpretation of dreams. In J. Strachey (Ed.), *The Standard Edition of the Complete Psychological Works of Sigmund Freud*, Volume IV. London: Hogarth Press.

Freud, S. (1908). Creative writers and daydreaming. In J. Strachey (Ed.), *The Standard Edition of the Complete Psychological Works of Sigmund Freud*, Volume IX (pp. 143–153). London: Hogarth Press.

Freud, S. (1915). Thoughts for the times on war and death. In J. Strachey (Ed.), *The Standard Edition of the Complete Psychological Works of Sigmund Freud*, Volume XIV (pp. 273–301). London: Hogarth Press.

Freud, S. (1917). Mourning and melancholia. In J. Strachey (Ed.), *The Standard Edition of the Complete Psychological Works of Sigmund Freud*, Volume XIV (pp. 237–258). London: Hogarth Press.

Freud, S. (1923). The ego and the id. In J. Strachey (Ed.), *The Standard Edition of the Complete Psychological Works of Sigmund Freud*, Volume XIX (pp. 1–66). London: Hogarth Press.

Freud, S. (1985). *The Complete Letters of Sigmund Freud and Wilhelm Fliess 1887–1904*. J. M. Masson (Ed.). Cambridge, MA: Harvard University Press.

Freud, S., & Abraham, K. (2002). *The Complete Correspondence of Sigmund Freud and Karl Abraham 1907–1925*. E. Falzeder (Ed.). London: Karnac.

Freud, S., & Binswanger, L. (2001). *The Freud-Binswanger Correspondence 1908–1938*. G. Fichtner (Ed.). New York: Other Press.

Freud, S., & Ferenczi, S. (1996). *The Correspondence of Sigmund Freud and Sandor Ferenczi*, Volume 2, 1914–1919. E. Falzeder & E. Brabant (Eds.). Cambridge, MA: Harvard University Press.

Gorer, G. (1965). *Death, Grief and Mourning*. New York: Doubleday.

Healy, D. (1997). *The Anti-Depressant Era*. Cambridge, MA: Harvard University Press.

Horn, L. (1989). *A Natural History of Negation*. Chicago: Chicago University Press.

Jackson, S. (1986). *Melancholia and Depression*. New Haven: Yale University Press.

Jacobson, E. (1954a). Contribution to the metapsychology of psychotic identifications. *Journal of the American Psychoanalytic Association, 2*, 239–262.

Jacobson, E. (1954b). Transference problems in the psychoanalytic treatment of severely depressive patients. *Journal of the American Psychoanalytic Association, 2*, 595–606.

Kaltenbeck, F. (2002). *Ce que Joyce etait pour Lacan*. Unpublished manuscript.

Klein, M. A (1935). Contribution to the psychogenesis of manic-depressive states. In *Love, Guilt and Reparation*. London: Hogarth, 1975.

Klein, M.A. (1940). Mourning and its relation to manic-depressive states. In M. Money-Kyrle (Ed.), *Love, Guilt and Reparation*. London: Hogarth, 1975.

Klein, M.A. (1952). Some theoretical conclusions regarding the emotional life of the infant. In *Envy and Gratitude* (pp. 61–93). London: Hogarth, 1975.

Lacan, J. (1958–59). *Le Désir et son Interpretation*. Unpublished seminar.

Lacan, J. (1959–60). *L'Ethique de la Psychanalyse*. J.-A. Miller (Ed.). Paris: Seuil, 1986.

Lacan, J. (1966). *Ecrits*. Paris: Seuil.

Lacan, J. (1974). *Television*. Paris: Seuil.

Lacan, J. (1991). *Le Séminaire. Livre VIII: Le Transfert*. J.-A. Miller (Ed.). Paris: Seuil, 1991.

Lacan, J. (1992). *The Seminar. Book VII: The Ethics of Psychoanalysis* (translated by D. Porter). J.-A. Miller (Ed.). New York and London: Routledge.

Lacan, J. (1994). *Le Séminaire. Livre IV: La Relation d'Objet*. J.-A. Miller (Ed.). Paris: Seuil, 1994.

Lacan, J. (2014). *The Seminar Book X: Anxiety* (translated by A.R. Price). J.-A. Miller (Ed.) Cambridge: Polity.

Laurent, E. (1988). Melancolie, douleur d'exister, lachete morale. *Ornicar? 47*, 5–17.

Little, M. (1986). *Transference Neurosis and Transference Psychosis: Towards Basic Unity*. London: Free Association Books.

Malcom, J. (1993). *The Silent Woman*. London: Papermac, 1995.

Menard, A. (1982). Sur le deuil et la melancolie. *Analytica, 29*, 47–61.

Metcalf, P., & Huntington, R. (1991). *Celebrations of Death* (3rd. ed.). Cambridge: Cambridge University Press.

Morel, G. (Ed.). (2002). *Clinique du Suicide*. Paris: Eres.

Owens, J. (1972). Metaphysical separation in Aquinas. *Medieval Studies*, *34*(1), 287–306.

Paskauskas, A. (Ed.) (1993). *The Complete Correspondence of Sigmund Freud and Ernest Jones 1908–1939*. Cambridge MA & London: Belknap Press of Harvard University Press.

Pellion, F. (2000). *Melancolie et verite*. Paris: Presses Universitaires de France, 2000.

Pollock, G. (1961). Mourning and adaptation. *International Journal of Psychoanalysis*, *42*, 341–371.

Pollock, G. (1970). Anniversary reactions, trauma, and mourning. *Psychoanalytic Quarterly*, *39*, 347–371.

Radden, J. (1987). Melancholy and melancholia. In D. M. Levin (Ed.), *Pathologies of the Modern Self* (pp. 231–50). New York: New York University Press.

Radden, J. (Ed.). (2000). *The Nature of Melancholy*. Oxford: Oxford University Press.

Roseman, M. (1999). Surviving memory: Truth and inaccuracy in Holocaust testimony. *Journal of Holocaust Education*, *8*, 1–20.

Roseman, M. (2000). *The Past in Hiding*. London: Penguin.

Rosenfeld, H. (1959). An investigation into the psycho-analytic theory of depression. *International Journal of Psychoanalysis*, *40*, 105–129.

Seaford, R. (1994). *Reciprocity and Ritual*. Oxford: Clarendon.

Segal, H. (1952). A psychoanalytic approach to aesthetics. In *The Work of Hanna Segal* (pp. 185–205). London: Free Association Books, 1986.

Schmidt, R. (1960). L'emploi de la separation en metaphysique. *Revue Philosophique de Louvain*, *58*, 373–393.

Spitz, R. (1960). Discussion of Dr. John Bowlby's paper, *Psychoanalytic Study of the Child*, *15*, 85–94.

Turnheim, M. (1997). Deuil et amour. *La Cause Freudienne*, *35*, 66–71.

Uspensky, B. (1973). *A Poetics of Composition*. Berkeley: University of California Press.

Vereecken, C., & Berge, A. E. (1993–1994). *L'Ideal du moi dans la nevrose obsessionnelle et dans la melancolie*. Oostende: Huize Louise-Marie.

Vereecken, C. (1986). Melancolie, perversion et identifications ideales. *Actes de L'Ecole de la Cause Freudienne*, *XI*, 24–29.

Vereecken, C. (1986). De la melancolie anxieuse aux fureurs heroiques. *Actes de L'Ecole de la Cause Freudienne'*, *XII*, 55–58.

Volkan, V. (1981). *Linking Objects and Linking Phenomena*. Madison: International Universities Press.

Wisdom, J. O. (1962). Comparison and development of the psychoanalytical theories of melancholia', *International Journal of Psycho-Analysis*, *43*, 113–132.

Wolfenstein, M. (1966). How is mourning possible? *Psychoanalytic Study of the Child*, *21*, 93–123.

Wright, E. (1999). *Speaking Desires Can Be Dangerous*. Oxford: Polity.

Zetzel, E. (1953). The depressive position. In *The Capacity for Emotional Growth* (pp. 63–81). London: Maresfield Reprints.

Chapter 5

Conceptualizing and treating (manic-depressive) psychosis

A Lacanian perspective

Stijn Vanheule

Lacanian psychoanalysis has a precise hypothesis about psychosis by assuming that psychosis makes up a *structure*. The hypothesis of a psychotic structure is not the only, or ultimate conceptual tool that Lacan and later Lacanian analysts use, but it is a crucial point of departure. For example, Lacan's later work focuses on psychosis *qua* a *jouissance*-related position or drive-related problem, as well as a particular way of creating psychical reality, largely conceptualized through mathematical knot theory. However, in this paper, I will concentrate on the hypothesis of structure and only briefly touch upon these later elaborations.[1] My key reference is Lacan's paper 'On a Question Prior to Any Possible Treatment of Psychosis' (1959).

The hypothesis of structure orients Lacanian practice and is quite precise. It does not imply that psychosis is an essence underlying the symptoms and acts of our patients, like a core biological or psychological constitution. Structure, by contrast, concerns how an individual represents him- or herself *via* language, and manages, or fails, to be constituted as a subject. With respect to language, Lacan particularly focuses on the signifier which is the elementary building block of language. The linguistic signs we use are signifiers to the extent that they do not have a strict signified or meaning. Meaning related to signifiers is context-dependent (Lacan, 1955–1956).

What is crucial concerning Lacan's point concerning the subject, is that at the level of the unconscious questions related to existence are formulated. In line with the Nietzschean dictum that man is a sick animal, Lacan assumes that the determination of human functioning by biology or by environmental factors is marked by a fundamental lack. His work on the mirror stage makes this clear (Lacan, 1949; 1961): natural maturation and instinctual patterns only partly determine who we are, thus leaving us, at the level of being, with an unpleasurable need, called the lack-of-being or want-to-be (*manqué-à-être*). "Organic discord", says Lacan (1959, p. 461), necessitates a "symbiosis with the Symbolic". Indeed, in dealing with the *Unbehagen* at the level of being, we make use of words or signifiers and live in terms of what culture and social contexts define as good. By using the signifier, and naming our own position with the personal pronoun, our precarious lack-of-being is turned into an articulated question of existence. However,

DOI: 10.4324/9781003216391-6

the *Other*, *qua* system of signifiers, and the *other*, *qua* interpersonal figure, only provide a partial answer to our want-to-be.

Fundamental self-directed *epistemic* questions ('who am I?') and questions concerning the *intentionality* of the other ('what do you want?') are never fully resolved. Instead, they set up a fundamental experience of dis-order and mobilize existential dilemmas which Lacan (1959) situates at the core of the unconscious. More specifically, he points out that the unconscious is organized around a set of existence-related questions or dilemmas, which no signifier can answer conclusively. These questions concern one's position with respect to intimate topics (see: Lacan, 1959, pp. 459, 461, 464), like:

1. Dealing with parenthood and authority – who am I as a child in relation to my parents and who am I as a parent in relation to my child?
2. Life in the light of death;
3. Sexuality in relation to love and procreation;
4. Sexuation – that is, the question as to whether, or how, one is a man or a woman.

Daily life confronts us with these issues, and, while no signifier can conclusively determine our identity, the stories we tell and the thoughts we have bear witness to the human attempt to resolve the vacillating position we occupy at the level of existence. What is more, this vacillation, as brought to the fore in our use of the signifier *vis-à-vis* questions related to existence, determines the subject.

From birth on, we see other people around us, and, through self-reflexivity, we are aware of the fact that we 'are'. We 'see' these points of lack-of-being. We not only see them: they are issues to us because we lack an automatic answer. Answers have to be formulated, and in the very process of articulating such answers, different structural possibilities might be discerned (Lacan, 1959). Crucial in this context is Lacan's distinction between neurosis and psychosis. These make up different structures because they imply a different way of dealing with the lack-of-being.

The Lacanian symptom

Many students who first read Lacan complain that his works are cruelly complex, yet this does not imply the assumption that all human beings are existentialist intellectuals who spend all night discussing and reflecting on the nature of human intentionality and identity. Not at all. Lacan (1959) hypothesizes that it is in and around symptoms that specific ways of dealing with the lack-of-being are expressed. Indeed, the way we deal with human intentionality and identity is to be situated at the level of the unconscious.

This is why, in Lacanian practice, much attention goes to discerning the crucial symptoms a patient is confronted with and studying how mental suffering is related to self-directed *epistemic* questions ('who am I?') and questions concerning the *intentionality* of the other ('what do you want?').

This approach implies that the Lacanian project goes radically against the way that the Diagnostic and Statistical Manual of Mental Disorders (DSM) approaches the symptom (Vanheule, 2017). The DSM takes symptoms for granted and classifies them as psychotic based on *a priori* grounds: the manual proposes a list of predefined psychotic symptoms and, if a patient's symptom sufficiently resembles these predefined symptoms, he is psychotic. By contrast, in Lacanian psychoanalysis, the symptom has no face value: we never know what it implies. It is only by listening to the patient's stories about the origin, nature, and contextual embedment of the symptom that we might get hold of the broader structure it bears witness to – that is, the psychotic structure.

In his 1959 paper, Lacan (p. 465) argues that, in neurosis, the question pertaining to the intentionality of the other is addressed in terms of a lawful principle, which is presumed at the basis of the other's actions. Indeed, in the clinical structure of neurosis, the subject takes shape starting from the belief that the other's actions are not random but guided by meaningful principles: social and cultural laws determine what the other does or should do. Lacan calls this lawful principle the, or a, 'Name-of-the-Father'. Starting from this signifier, which is accepted in neurosis, sense can be made of the 'desire-of-the-mother'. Considered from the angle of the Name-of-the-Father the (m)other is a fairly regulated entity that one can rely upon. Hence, for example, the experience of disappointment, anger, or shame in neurosis, when others don't live up to the expectations imposed onto them.

In psychosis, by contrast, a Name-of-the-Father is radically missing. It is foreclosed, says Lacan (1959, pp. 465–466; Grigg, 2008). A Name-of-the-Father, or a master signifier, is a signifier that is taken for granted and a means by which the subject can manifest itself at the moment one is presumed to take a position in relation to the Other, or in relation to the questions related to existence that make up the unconscious. A Name-of-the-Father is a signifier in the name of which one speaks and takes a position *vis-à-vis* the Other. For example, imagine a father with a young toddler. At times, the child says nasty things like "nanny is wee wee". At such a point the father might intervene and tell his son to behave. Yet, typically, toddlers don't obey when one says this, which might bring the father to say something like: "you have to stop doing this because daddy says so". In this example, the signifier "daddy" is a Name-of-the-Father. It is a signifier in the name of which the parent positions himself and guides the child.

What is characteristic of psychosis is that at specific events in a life, which typically involve others, the subject fails to make use of, or find, such a master signifier, or Name-of-the-Father to represent him- or herself in relation to these questions pertaining to existence. The net result of such a confrontation is that one no longer experiences continuity at the level of mental life: the subject collapses and an experience of crisis accompanied by intrusive symptoms comes to the fore.

Lacanian theory assumes that we experience continuity at the level of mental life because we have signifiers or representations by means of which we make sense of the world (Lacan, 1957). For example, when giving a lecture, I'm not perplexed by the fact that people are staring at me, and occasionally whisper into each other's ear, because I have a conceptual frame through which I can make sense of what is happening; I have such a parameter because I trust or accept that the signifier 'lecturing' names and organizes what is happening in the room. Thanks to the signifier, 'lecturing', I can situate myself as 'speaker' and the others as 'audience', which organizes my mental representations.

Within this logic, when do basic manifestations of psychotic structure come to the fore? That will be when an appeal to position oneself *via* the signifier is made, but no support is found in any signifier, which interrupts the signifying chain, or train of thoughts, that make up our experience of reality. Lacan's structural idea concerning psychosis implies the hypothesis that foreclosure pertaining to questions related to existence at the level of unconscious determines the outbreak of specific psychotic phenomena.

This means that, because of such confrontations, psychotic phenomena such as hallucinations, delusions, or mental automatism might come to the fore. Clinically, these phenomena all concern being overwhelmed by strange experiences one cannot make sense of, and bear witness to a more fundamental inability to manifest oneself as a subject using the signifier.

Specifically, mental automatism concerns an often-subtle experience of disarraying interruption occurring in the continuity of how a person experiences him-/herself and/or the world. As he explains in his third seminar, Lacan (1955–1956) borrowed this concept from the early 20th-century French psychiatrist, Gaëtan Gatian de Clérambault. Suddenly, or gradually over time, one's own thoughts, utterances, emotions, impulses, actions, and bodily sensations come across as disordered in nature. On the one hand, strange elements might be added to the habitual self-experience, where a feeling of being intruded upon stands to the fore. In that case, an invading 'parasitic' component destabilizes the subject. On the other hand, the interruption might also result from a blocking inhibition; one becomes deprived of what is familiar. In both cases, an experience of estrangement is produced: the coordinates from which one situates oneself in the world seem no longer valid. Empty-handed, the subject is confronted with fundamental changes at the heart of his privacy.

At that point, two possibilities come to the fore. Either one ends up utterly perplexed, in that the breach in the signifying chain is presented in all its rudeness. In that case, the signifying chain comes to a halt. Signifying articulation stops with a dead end, which will often be accompanied by the belief that the shadow of death has fallen onto one's life. The other possibility is that, instead of dying out, the signifying chain starts to function in uncontrolled ways, and thus alternative signifiers alluding to the failed naming resulting from foreclosure are produced in the subject's reality (Vanheule, 2011).

Clinically speaking, this implies that, upon encountering an elementary phenomenon in a patient's discourse, we have to construct, through case formulation, how mental automatism might be associated with specific events of failure in representing oneself by means of the signifier in relation to the Other.

What is specific to Lacan's account of mental automatism when compared to that of De Clérambault, which was purely mechanical, is that it enables us to grasp why psychotic symptoms touch on specific contents. Foreclosure implies that specific issues concerning sexuality, death, and human intentionality cannot be addressed in terms of any assumed law, which implies that the subject cannot manifest itself in an organized way. Yet this does not imply that these issues themselves would not be articulated. Far from it. These questions are manifested in particular ways, that is: in a Real way through automatic phenomena, which manifest in wild, unexpected, and brutal ways, and confront the subject with the contents that could not be assumed *via* a master signifier or Name-of-the-Father.

Hence, for example, Schreber's daydream that it must be beautiful to be a woman making love, which is an automatically imposed thought he, at least at first, cannot make sense of. The thought occurs to him at the moment he fails to assert his masculinity after losing the election for parliament. His masculinity collapses, and suddenly a feminizing thought overwhelms him.

Characteristically, the moment the ability to orient oneself as a subject by means of the signifier is absent, another more threatening position comes to take its place. This is the position of being the object of the other's *jouissance*. '*Jouissance*' is the French word for enjoyment and makes up a typical Lacanian concept. Lacan (1970) preferred to continue using the French word '*jouissance*' in English translations of his work. The reason for this is that 'enjoyment' refers too strongly to amusement and gratification, while Lacan uses the concept to refer to a kind of enjoyment that is not bound to the pleasure principle. Usually, one does not experience *jouissance* as an agent. Rather, it is an internal or external force that takes one by surprise. In neurosis, *jouissance* is limited by a Name-of-the-Father. In psychosis, by contrast, it occasionally overwhelms the subject completely since foreclosure leaves no anchorage in the Symbolic order.

Take the case of Aimée, which is the central case study in Lacan's (1932) doctoral dissertation. This patient fails to occupy a mothering position in relation to her son, and suddenly she thinks that people want to hurt her baby, which indicates that she occupies a position in which she is the object of the other's *jouissance*. In her case, this not only results in distrust but also in violent acts towards people she doesn't trust. These violent acts (called *passage-à-l'actes*) function as attempts to limit *jouissance* in the Real when the Symbolic provides no protection anymore (see also: Leader, 2011).

Lacanian rehabilitation

This theory has profound implications for clinical practice. In the case of neurosis, we assume that symptoms express ambivalence, conflict, and repression concerning the signifiers mobilized in addressing the questions of existence at the level of the unconscious. Therapy consists of analyzing such conflict by means of free association, which leads to recognizing elements that have first been repressed by means of a Name-of-the-Father or master signifier, and eventually to a different attitude towards desire and towards the question as to how one should deal with *jouissance*.

In psychosis, by contrast, there is no guiding Name-of-the-Father or master signifier. What is more, upon confrontations with questions of existence at the level of the unconscious through situations in daily life, no signifier is there to represent the subject, and as a result, all subjective order is lost. The Other goes mad. Nevertheless, the psychotic structure does not imply that *all* confrontations with self-related epistemic questions, or questions pertaining to the intentionality of the other, invariably lead to elementary phenomena, hallucinations, or delusions. Rather, it implies that, if there are psychotic symptoms, the psychoanalyst should examine whether, and how, through specific events and situations in life, the psychotic crisis was triggered.

Metaphorically speaking, neurotic symptoms are displaced signifiers that appear in unexpected contexts, and as a result, to paraphrase Freud (1919), they provoke the feeling that one is not the master in one's own house. Psychotic experiences, by contrast, come with perplexity, and, often, also with dismay. They are manifestations of unthinkable or unimaginable signifiers, with which one, at least initially, feels no link. However, given that such invading signifiers interfere within the signifying chain that constitutes the subject, they cannot simply be put aside. By this imposition of a strange element amid how I approach the world, such parasitic signifiers undermine the identity I experience of myself and of others. To use Freud's metaphor, they destabilize the idea of having a haven that protects us against the world outside. Psychotic experiences are bombs that (threaten to) make the house explode or implode.

The psychoanalytic treatment of psychosis aims at running counter to this tendency. In this respect, it could be argued that the Lacanian treatment of psychosis *par excellence* aims at *rehabilitation*. Etymologically, 'rehabilitation' is rooted in the Latin word '*habitare*', which means to inhabit. Lacanian psychoanalysis aims at finding and inventing tailor-made solutions that make the house of mental life and social relations inhabitable again. Obviously, such 'Lacanian rehabilitation' is far removed from adapting individuals to societal norms and standards. It aims at finding singular solutions for experiences that threaten and undermine the subject.

Practically, this implies that we don't aim at installing free association. After all, repression is not an issue in psychosis. The position the analyst takes is different and aims at helping the subject find an answer in response to perplexing or maddening situations. This response might be diverse. It could consist of finding an identification to believe in, developing a habit or practice to hold on to, or formulating a rule to adhere to. Structurally, the answer we must invent by means of psychoanalytic work, at least temporarily, fills the gap of foreclosure. In his later work, Lacan calls such a private solution that creates stability in mental life a 'sinthome' (see also Vanheule, 2011). 'Sinthome' is the more ancient spelling of 'symptom' (Lacan, 1975–1976), and although Lacan switches between both terms, the concept of sinthome specifically refers to ways of dealing with *jouissance* that create stability in mental life. One reason why Lacan switches to the word sinthome is that it has interesting equivocal connotations. 'Sinthome' plays on the English word 'sin' and on the French phrase '*saint homme*', which means 'saintly man', and refers to the person who does the right thing. In Lacan's (1975–1976, p. 13) interpretation, a sinthome unites both dimensions: on the one hand, it refers to a person's 'sins', or frailties, and, on the other hand, it bears witness to a person's *savoir faire* in dealing with such frailties.

To conclude the theoretical part of my paper, I would now like to introduce a brief note on transference. In neurosis, transference implies that knowledge is attributed to the analyst, which, at the side of the analysand, leads to occupying a specific role, like the role of the one who always feels stupid because of knowing so little, or the role of the one who always ends up lying, and masking aspects of reality. In psychosis, by contrast, transference tends towards what Lacan (1966, p. 4) calls "mortifying erotomania" (see also: Leader, 2011). This means that, in transference, the patient threatens to end up feeling like a puppet in the hands of the analyst – that is, the object of the other's *jouissance*. Indeed, at the level of transference, foreclosure is expressed. If the patient fails to make sense of what it is that the analyst wants, or aims at, mortifying erotomania might come to the fore. Just as what is often the case outside treatment situations, the question concerning the intentionality of the Other presents in the treatment too. Whereas, in neurosis, aspects of analytical silence and the not-knowing position of the analyst safeguard the articulation of desire, these often have a reverse effect in psychosis. In psychosis, silence can fuel the conclusion that one is the target of the analyst's *jouissance*, meaning the object of how he or she, in an unregulated and limitless way, satisfies his or her drive. If such a conclusion comes to the fore, transference is a mere dual relation, in which the patient is delivered to an obscure and merciless other. Therefore, in clinical work, the analyst should aim at installing a triangular situation, which makes clear that the analyst's interventions are not guided by highly subjective impulses and preferences, but by a guiding rationale.

A clinical case

The following case discussion aims at indicating how the abstract Lacanian treatment principles might be translated clinically. The case concerns Marianne, a 46-year-old woman. Considered, from a psychiatric point of view, her symptoms fit with the syndrome of manic-depressive psychosis. She starts consulting me because of deep despair concerning several aspects of her life. I will address two issues she struggled with: the meaning of life after the death of her best friend Elisa, and the question of being a mother to her daughter.

First, a note on transference. In neurosis, the psychoanalytic setting is fixed, with free association and a characteristic style of responding by the analyst, in which silence plays an important role. The enigma of the analyst's presence fuels the analysand in exploring the enigma of her unconscious. In psychosis, such an enigmatic position is often threatening. It does not stimulate the articulation of the subject but rather confronts the analysand with the object-like position. Therefore, interventions are needed that convince the analysand that the position of the analyst is not an instance of *jouissance*, but rather a castrated position, to which the specific analyst the patient is working with is also subjected.

In my work with Marianne, from early in our sessions, she starts molding transference by imposing restraints on my habitual way of practicing. For example, she tells me that she cannot stand gazes she cannot see. For example, in a restaurant, she will never sit with her back to other people. She must see what other people are looking at. Usually, I let patients enter my office first, and I close the door. Marianne asks me to enter first so that she can close the door. Typically, I see people face to face while sitting in comfortable chairs. However, Marianne asks me if we can talk at my desk since she prefers to have a table between both of us. I agreed with both proposals since they impose a limit on how we will interact. At the level of speech itself, Marianne again intervenes. After a couple of sessions, Marianne asks me to ask more questions since silence fuels her despair, and, since then, I have taken more care in asking her questions when silences come to the fore. Silence does not accentuate her subjective division and uncertainty but does make her identify with the position of the abject object. In a similar vein, she asks me to start each session with a specific question, which is not something I would usually do. Again, I agree. The demands Marianne makes impose a limit and rule on my actions. Therefore, I agreed. This way of handling transference does not mean that one should always comply with each demand of an analysand.

From Marianne's very first session, her speech is most fluent. Speech runs on wheels, but the subjective effects are extreme. During the first year of our sessions, she regularly sends me e-mails after each session in which she indicates that her despair is enormous and that things at home make her mad. In neurosis, speech has truth-effects. Through speech, the subject is actualized. This means that speech itself, and the fact that the analysand hears both herself, and occasionally the analyst intervene, orients the analysand to acknowledge things that are true for her and to act likewise. Lacan expressed this as: "the spoken clarification is the mainspring of progress" (Lacan, 1954–1955, p. 255). In contrast, in psychosis, speech often does not have such a clarifying, orienting, and pacifying effect. Rather speech tends to actualize the very structure of what led to the production of situations of distress and psychotic outbreaks. This does not mean that we should automatically refrain from talking therapy, but rather that, through talking therapy, solutions must be found that counter foreclosure. Psychoanalytic treatment aims at finding limits in relation to the unlimited *jouissance* coming to the fore when speech addresses psychotic phenomena and/or topics at the level of which foreclosure is playing; limits that help the analysand to avoid the position of being the object in the claws of an unpredictable and/or merciless other.

During the therapy, Marianne finds two kinds of limits. First, an aspect of her story that is maddening for her is silenced when she gets tattooed with a self-designed image that refers to that aspect of her story – i.e., once the tattoo, to which she connects a condensed story, is on her body, she stops talking about that issue. At the start of our therapy, she has one tattoo. After two years of therapy, four tattoos were added to her body. With each tattoo, the memory is suddenly 'on hold'. In terms of Lacanian theory, these tattoos function as holophrases that have a sinthomatic value and bring consistency to mental life. Second, maddening aspects of her daily life become more manageable when I provide her with ideas through which she can reflect on situations at home.

First, let me explore a tattoo example. Marianne and Elisa meet during an evening class in French. The students have to do an exercise in pairs, and they accidentally end up together. It is the encounter of her life. Marianne and Elisa become best friends. She has never before met a person like Elisa. They understand each other completely and talk about everything, except sex. At that time, Marianne is married and has two children. Soon, Elisa joins the household and helps Marianne with the kids. Around that time, Marianne gives birth to a third child, and both women take care of the baby. Some months later, Elisa starts dating a man. She joins him on a business trip and, tragically, they have a car accident on a snowy road, and they both die. Since then, Marianne's world collapses. She says that Elisa had even asked her if she should stay with her and the kids instead of going on the trip, but Marianne said she should go. Upon telling this story Marianne is filled with despair: nothing makes sense in life, and she sees no way out of her misery. Elisa was Marianne's double, her '*doppelgänger*'. Upon losing her, she loses herself and invariably concludes that since Marianne's death she is worthless. Before starting therapy, these experiences of despair regularly gave rise to risk-seeking behavior simulating Elisa's death, like racing on highways. During therapy, such passages stop.

This story provides the basis of two tattoos. The first one is a dragon. She says that it refers to Chinese mythology and symbolizes the connection with the dead. Once the tattoo is there, Marianne is somewhat pacified. She proudly shows the tattoo and goes on discussing other topics. In contrast with what happens in therapy with neurosis, speech does not lead to attributing a different place to herself and Elisa, or to reconsider their relationship. The tattoo is a sign of their mythical close bond; a sign that seems to reassure her that, maybe, not all concerning Elisa is lost.

Next to that, maddening aspects of daily life become more manageable when I provide her with ideas through which she can reflect on situations at home. Currently, Marianne has six children. When she starts consulting me, her only daughter had just started attending elementary school at the age of six. Before that she didn't attend school; Marianne couldn't stand the idea that her daughter would be away from her. Now, because of school attendance laws, Marianne must take a distance, which frightens her. At the same time, she cannot adequately take care of her daughter: when she was born, Marianne couldn't wash or feed the baby or change her diapers. She was afraid that touching the child would have a traumatic impact. Now, Marianne does not know how to make sure that her daughter arrives at school on time and therefore stays in bed, and, as a result, she feels guilt and starts to blame herself. I wonder aloud if the older sons could maybe assist. Marianne is surprised by the suggestion, but indeed asks the older sons to take care of their sister in the morning, which goes quite well. As a result, Marianne can now wake up with her children in the morning and have breakfast with them.

The Lacanian treatment of psychosis starts from the assumption that at the level of the unconscious, some themes cannot be addressed in a steady way. A lawful Name-of-the-Father is missing. Therefore, alternative ways of naming or handling the issues that bear witness to foreclosure need to be invented. In Marianne's case, foreclosure concerns the question of being a mother in relation to her children. As she meets Elisa, Marianne seems to enter a world of magical connectedness, which turns the question of raising children into something self-evident. How she experienced it before meeting Elisa is unclear. Yet, with Elisa's death, this changes dramatically. Suddenly, nothing is self-evident anymore and Marianne ends up in a melancholic position. During therapy, Marianne first starts rebuilding her own imaginary identity. Tattooing helps her to stop thinking about painful events from the past. What first marked her subjectively is now marked on her body. These tattoos are so-called *sinthomatic* solutions (Miller, 2001) by means of which Marianne avoids falling into the hole of nonsense that foreclosure opened in her existence. Next to that, during the consultations she finds ideas around which she can raise her children. Situations at home still provoke distress, but their effect on her is less devastating.

Note

1 For broader discussions of Lacan's conceptualization of psychosis, see: Leader, 2011; Vanheule, 2011.

References

Freud, S. (1955 [1919]). The "Uncanny". In *The Complete Psychological Works*, Vol. XVII, pp.217–256. London: Hogarth Press.

Grigg, R. (2008). *Lacan, Language and Philosophy*. Albany: State University of New York Press.

Lacan, J. (1932). *De la Psychose Paranoïaque dans ses Rapports avec la Personnalité*. Paris: Seuil.

Lacan, J. (2006 [1949]). The Mirror Stage as Formative of the Function of the I' in J. Lacan and J.A. Miller (eds.) *Écrits*, pp. 75–81. New York and London: W. W. Norton.

Lacan, J. (1993 [1955–56]). *The Seminar 1955–1956, Book III, The Psychoses*. New York and London: W.W. Norton.

Lacan, J. (2006 [1957]). The Instance of the Letter in the Unconscious or Reason since Freud. In J. Lacan and J.A. Miller (eds.) *Écrits*, pp. 412–442. New York and London: W. W. Norton.

Lacan, J. (2006 [1959]). On a Question Prior to Any Possible Treatment of Psychosis. In J. Lacan and J.A. Miller (eds.) *Écrits*, pp. 445–488. New York and London: W. W. Norton.

Lacan, J., (1966). Presentation of the Memoirs of president Schreber in French translation. *Analysis*, 7, 1–4.

Lacan, J. (2005 [1975–76]). *Le séminaire 1975–1976, Livre XXIII, Le Sinthome*. Paris: Seuil.

Leader, D. (2011). *What Is Madness?* London: Hamish Hamilton.

Miller, J.A. (2001). L'orientation lacanienne III, Le lieu et le lien. *La Cause Freudienne*, 48, 7–35.

Vanheule, S. (2011). *The Subject of Psychosis: A Lacanian Perspective*. London & New York: Palgrave Macmillan.

Vanheule, S. (2017). *Psychiatric Diagnosis Revisited: From DSM to Clinical Case Formulation*. London & New York: Palgrave Macmillan.

Chapter 6

Maneuvers of transference in psychosis

A case study of melancholia from a Lacanian perspective

Joachim Cauwe and Stijn Vanheule

The handling of transference is central to psychoanalytic practice. In this chapter, we examine how therapeutic work can be approached in psychosis, starting from the specific nature of psychotic transference through the detailed discussion of a case from our practice.

The work of Lacan pertaining to psychosis specifically can be divided into several eras (Vanheule, 2011). Lacan is best known for his interpretation of Freudian psychoanalysis through a focus on the Symbolic, unraveling how linguistic mechanisms structure psychic experience. With regard to psychosis, specifically, foreclosure of the Name-of-the-Father (Facchin, 2016; Vanheule, 2011) was the crucial concept for the classical Lacan. The theory on foreclosure describes how in psychosis a conventional reference point to answer questions of existence is absent. Imagine that one is observing a game of boules, but without seeing the little ball (the '*cochonnet*' or piglet) that is central to determining strategy and the primary factor as to who wins or loses the game. One sees the players celebrating, getting excited, and anxious, but without having a mental schema to interpret these reactions. It takes a lot of thinking and theorizing to come up with ideas that can somewhat frame these enigmatic interactions. The deficit correlative of foreclosure has to do with the Symbolic ('the rules of the game'), against the background of intact cognitive capacities. We can often observe how in psychosis the patient is working very hard to make sense of reality and others (trying to deduce the rules that might govern the game). Lacan relates the lacking symbolic element in foreclosure to psychotic phenomena and ways of relating to others observed in the clinic.

However, during the 1960s, Lacan became increasingly interested in experiences beyond the limits of language; conceptually, Lacan developed the 'object *a*' and '*jouissance*' to reflect on these limits (Vanheule, 2011). The concepts of object *a* and *jouissance*[1] are approached in different ways throughout the development of Lacan's seminars. We will situate them through Lacan's discussion in seminar X ('*Anxiety*'), where they emerge as central concepts in thinking about analytic experience and transference specifically. Then, we will outline the way this perspective influences how transference and psychosis (and their conjunction) are approached.

DOI: 10.4324/9781003216391-7

Jouissance and object *a* in seminar **X**: the schema of subjective division

Seminar X questions the borders of signification, the core idea being that certain aspects of mental experience cannot be expressed through language. As a result, it is generally considered a tipping point in his oeuvre. Whereas the subject is supported by the signifier (Figure 6.1) (linguistic elements), Lacan (1962–1963) uses the letter '*a*' to denote 'what resists any assimilation to the function of a signifier' (p. 174). First, we turn to the schema of subjective division, put forward in that seminar, as it outlines the role of the *object a* in the transformation of the subject of *jouissance* and the emergence of a desiring subject, which he indicates by barring the letter S: $.

Lacan describes the dialectical relation between the subject and the Other ('A' for 'Autre'). The schema (Figure 1) represents the side of the Other on the left and that of the subject on the right. In the first logical step (top of Figure 1), there is a 'subject of *jouissance*' (p. 173) in the constitution of desire: it is a mythical subject that is devoid of any lack (hence, it is indicated by a capital S, in contrast to the barred S that appears at the lower level of Lacan's scheme). This 'primordial subject' (p. 173) has to 'realize himself on the path to the Other' (p. 173). This operation is discussed by Lacan as following a long division; through this operation of division, a remainder is produced ('*a*') that cannot be taken up by the Other of language. However, because this leftover is situated in the field of the Other in neurosis, it is at the same time a 'port of access' (p. 179) to the Other. This makes possible a translation of *jouissance* to the plane of desire. Whereas *jouissance* is a solitary enjoyment, that cannot be expressed or shared, desire establishes a connection to the Other.

We now turn to the consequences of this extraction for neurotic desire and transference, then we describe the consequences of non-extraction in psychosis in the following section. Desire, for Lacan, emerges against the background of loss; something from the original mythical *jouissance*, a part of the body ('a pound of flesh', p. 124), has to be lost, for a subject to be able to desire: this is the case in neurosis, where *jouissance* and the Other meet in fantasy. The object *a* thus indicates the missing piece of the puzzle that is fantasized to be in the Other in neurosis. It becomes the cause of desire and puts the subject in a position of lack in relation to the Other. In seminar VIII (*Transference*), Lacan linked this aspect of the relation to the Other with the ancient Greek term 'agalma' (Lacan, 1960 – 61, p. 167), a hidden treasure or small deity. Following a reflection on love, based on Plato's symposium, love is conceptualized as the assumption that this brilliant agalma is lodged in the Other, and Lacan states that transference

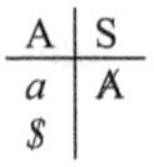

$$
\begin{array}{c|c}
A & S \\
\hline
a & \bar{A} \\
\$ &
\end{array}
$$

Figure 6.1 The schema of subjective division (based on Lacan, 1962–63, p. 160)

is possible because of this. To be more specific, the enigmatic presence of the analyst is a motor force to set speech in motion (Cauwe, Vanheule & Desmet, 2017). In neurosis, the subject goes on a quest for this (forever) missing piece in and through the Other. The 'possibility of transference' (Lacan 1962–1963, p. 337), then, comes down to situating the *a,* as such, in the field of the Other. In neurosis, what has been lost is situated and looked for in the Other. Loss enables desire, the cause of which is fantasized to be in the Other.

Thus far, we have discussed that desire in neurosis is possible according to Lacan because of a loss that occurs when the subject meets the Other of language. As a consequence of this extraction, *jouissance* becomes regulated through fantasy.

Crazy in love: psychotic transference from the perspective of object *a* and *jouissance*

From the perspective of narcissism, Freud (1914) considered that in cases of psychosis, libido is not attached to objects because all libido is withdrawn from the outside world and invested in the ego. However, for an analytic process to be possible, the analyst has to become a libidinal object so that transference can develop. However, it has now been well established that Freud was wrong about the capacity for transference in psychosis.

Lacan progressively put forward the dimension of the object in his reflection on analysis and transference, which begs the question of how this outlook on the object affects his reflections on psychosis.

From a Lacanian perspective, psychosis is marked by the non-separation of the object *a*. According to Lacan, 'the psychotic has the object in his pocket' (Lacan, 1967, as cited in: Maleval, 2015, p. 103). This has two important consequences that directly impact the therapeutic work with psychosis. First, *jouissance* is not limited through loss as in neurosis but imposes itself in an unregulated fashion on the psychotic patient. *Jouissance* refers here to an overwhelming non-signified excitation that manifests itself from within (Vanheule, 2011, p. 137).

Secondly, transference bears witness to an inverted structure, based on the will of the Other. In neurosis, object *a* is situated on the side of the Other and acts as a support of fantasy; based on a faith in the Other, the neurotic patient can question his existence through the Symbolic. In psychosis, a fundamentally skeptical and distant attitude towards the Other is present; the Other's rules and explanations are not trusted as a benchmark for addressing questions of desire (Vanheule, 2011, p. 136). The thesis of the non-separation of the object *a* clarifies the structure of the relation to the Other (and hence, transference) in psychosis; rather than looking for the missing piece to satisfy an intrinsically unsatiable desire through fantasy, as in neurosis, psychosis is marked by the reverse: the Other looks for something in the patient. Lacan (1966, p. 217) used the term '*érotomanie morti-fiante*',[2] mortifying erotomania, to denote an aspect of transference whereby the patient is put in the degrading position of being the object of someone's exclusive attention. The reference to erotomania means that Lacan considered psychotic transference from the perspective of the psychotic experience of knowing that the Other is interested in the subject and totally invested in its existence. There is no veil covering the Other's desire nor is there a position of questioning what it is that causes this desire, as in neurosis. Psychotic transference is marked by the experience of an Other that is either madly in love with, or has a profound hatred for, the subject; this love or hate is boundless and encompassing. The patient can thus experience him/herself to be the object (*jouissance*) of the Other. This is most evident in the case of paranoia, where the patient is persecuted by others (e.g., being spied on by a colleague). Psychosis is characterized by the experience that the Other has gone mad. Intimate relations can pose serious problems because of the excessive interest of the Other; often, in psychosis, anxiety or intrusive phenomena are experienced following an erotic or romantic encounter and unmediated intimacy can be possibly perplexing, threatening, and anxiety-inducing. A therapeutic relationship (in most forms of psychotherapy) also automatically implies this intimacy (because of the context and content of psychotherapy sessions), thus possibly inducing similar processes.

Transference in psychosis raises the question of how analysts can position themselves to avoid becoming a mortifying presence. Lacan raised this question of 'the maneuver of transference'[3], (Lacan, 1959, p. 583), in his text 'On a question prior to any possible treatment of psychosis'. The analyst has to lend herself to different uses, depending on the singularity and structural features of the patient that she is faced with. If the treatment process is marked by a neurotic dynamic, the analyst becomes a (symbolic) representative of the Other; the patient can question the desire of the analyst but is not directly confronted with her *jouissance*. Transference is triangular, with the patient having the supposition that the process of analysis will result in the acquisition of lacking knowledge about his or her functioning, leading the patient to search for knowledge from the analyst and in the analytic process. Analysis is a treatment through and with the Other, where the aspect of transference love motivates the production of meaning through free association. In Lacanian therapy, moreover, neurotic patients are invited to accept responsibility for their own contribution to the suffering they complain of. Lacan (1951) discussed this aspect of subjective involvement through the Dora case, where Freud pointed out to Dora that she was an active organizer of the situation she complained about in analysis, by helping out with the kids of frau K. so that her father could have his way with frau K.

In psychotic transference, because of the inherent tendency of a dual relation, the analyst cannot rely on her symbolic authority (as a stand-in for the Other) to regulate the therapeutic interaction as transference has an inverted form: the Other is interested in and transfers onto the patient (Zenoni, 2008). The initiative is on the side of the Other who wants something from the patient, who loves or hates the patient without limit; put differently, the Other is not castrated and appears without lack. Here, the treatment is that of the Other; as Silvestre (1984, cited in Maleval, 2015, p. 104) points out, the patient expects signifiers to organize his disordered world and offers his *jouissance* to be regulated by the analyst. Hence, maneuvers are interventions that limit invasive *jouissance* or try to give a name to troubling aspects of experience.

Often, indications on how to work with psychosis are based on injunctions to abstain from making Oedipal interpretations and interventions pointing to a 'hidden desire'; moreover, the focus is mostly on avoiding a dual relation. Nevertheless, when the clinician can avoid being in the position of an almighty and whimsical Other, the transferential tie with the clinician can become an important element in finding a balance and looking for solutions to what troubles psychotic patients. Speech in Lacanian-inspired therapy with psychotic patients can be characterized as a conversation, going from one topic to another with both partners exchanging listening and making their point(s); a dialogue somewhat akin to an everyday conversational context. This differs from work with neurotic patients, where the analyst is often more of a silent listener, supporting free association. However, in psychosis, an all-too-silent listener could risk inflating a dual relation where silence is experienced as malevolence or as a means of power.

In this chapter, we explore what maneuvering might be, through the description of psychotherapy with a man presenting with melancholic psychosis, based on Lacanian principles. Moreover, we pay special attention to the interventions aimed at keeping the transference manageable – specifically, avoiding the position of the Other without lack, by indicating how, as an analyst, we are also castrated and limited as subjects in a symbolic universe. Furthermore, we demonstrate how the mad Other can be interpreted. Finally, we outline how a partnership, centered on 'affinities', enabled this patient to have a more bearable life. The use of the term 'affinities' is inspired by Ron Suskind who coined the term 'affinity therapy' (Maleval & Grollier, 2017); he developed a way of communicating with his severely autistic and mute son through his son's passion for Disney figures. This approach is in line with psychoanalytic work with patients facing severe difficulties in social contexts; it centers on the passions, interests, and projects that the patient is drawn to. We want to demonstrate how the particularity of the psychotic position was encountered and dealt with in this singular encounter.

The patient was treated by the first author, who is a male psychotherapist trained using the Freudian-Lacanian perspective with which he practices. He had 7 years of experience working as a psychotherapist in settings with ambulatory patients and has a Ph.D. in clinical psychology. The case material covers the first year and a half of the treatment, conducted in private practice.

Case: Hans

Hans is a single man in his 50s, consulting because of a depressive mood that has been present for over a year. In the first consultation, Hans talked about how he has been feeling very depressed and sad over the last few months; he has been unemployed for over a year, ever since his last job ended. He is overwhelmed with sadness when asked about his studies or employment because he feels he has failed at both. He said that he used to enjoy sculpting and expressing himself creatively, but that recently he has been unable to engage in those activities for months on end. Moreover, his life has become a heavy burden and he is unable to experience joyful or satisfactory moments; the depressive mood and lack of pleasure had been especially pronounced during the last year. However, he has struggled with feelings of emptiness and anxiety throughout his life, which led to him being hospitalized multiple times for approximately 6 months each time. He was first hospitalized following very negative feedback during a course he took in high school. His last hospitalization was just 5 years ago, some months after his mother had passed away. Importantly, during this last stay in the hospital, Hans was able to speak about the loss of his mother; however, he was unable to utter a single word regarding his loss in the company of family members (so as not to burden his father any more than he already was). He felt he could talk about this in the hospital because people pointed out to him 'that it was a normal thing to grieve'.

When Hans lost his mother, it hit him very hard; he felt like he had lost the one person in the world whom he was certain would help him through any difficulty. Even though his mother was rather quiet, grumpy, and easily upset by any form of conflict or quarrel, Hans said she became more genial towards the end of her life. Nonetheless, her loss caused him to face severe difficulties in his life. In some sessions, he spoke of a dream he had about his mother, in which she was alive, but had disappeared.

Hans's father was characterized as a sad and anxious man who had been that way for as long as Hans could remember. Hans linked his father's disposition to the death of one of his father's siblings when Hans was just a few months old. Following this death, his father lost all enjoyment in life, and the familial atmosphere seemed to have been characterized by a permanent state of mourning. No one was now allowed to play music in the house, even though Hans and his mother loved music and enjoyed dancing together. Moreover, Hans recounted how every outburst of excitement from him, and his brother was always met with the sentence: 'it's going to end up in tears'.

Invasive *jouissance*: (melancholic) self-reproach, others, and the body

I worked with Hans from a diagnosis of psychosis, even though he did not experience positive symptoms (e.g., hallucinations or delusions) more broadly associated with psychosis[4]. As described above, psychosis is marked by a *jouissance* that is not regulated, because a limit is lacking due to the non-separation of the object *a*. Several aspects of Hans's discourse indicated how he was plagued by a *jouissance* that he was unable to put into words. Hans repeatedly stated that he had always been unable to express how bad he really felt; additionally, he struggled with what he called 'emptiness'. There were no words to express this incessantly reappearing 'bad' thing; feeling bad debilitated him to the point that there was nothing he could do to stop it and this excessive *jouissance* beyond words appeared in several ways.

First, what constituted the thread of Hans's life was the idea of his nullity; the idea that he was worthless and a burden to others was at the center of his experience of the world. Such constant self-deprecation, the relentless attacks on himself, is one of the core features of melancholia (Freud, 1917; Leader, 2008). Lacan renders the function of the relation to the image of the self in melancholia as follows in seminar X: 'Initially, he attacks this image so as to reach, within it, the object *a* that transcends him, whose control escapes him' (Lacan, 1962–1963, p. 335).

The 'ravaging' (Grigg, 2015, p. 144) object was not separated and continuously escaped Hans's control. Melancholia is characterized by a *jouissance* of self-hatred. Grigg (2015) proposes that an equivalent to the megalomanic 'I love myself' is to be found in the melancholic's 'I hate myself' (p. 141). In therapy, Hans talked about having no value for other people; he felt abandoned by most people in his life, including some close relatives: 'I couldn't bear to be around myself either, they are probably right in leaving me behind'. He said that he is a failure in life since he is unable to maintain a relationship with a partner and has no children. Several topical threads converged in the first sessions in a statement Hans made repeatedly: 'I must be a really difficult person'. He summed up a series of events to back up this statement, this final judgment of his being.

A second aspect where *jouissance* appeared was in his relationships with others. These relations were not structured around lack or conflict, as would be the case in neurosis, but rather demonstrated that the presence of others (both transferential and outside the transference) baffled him and posed great difficulties for him; he mostly perceived others as completely disinterested or whimsical. This constituted an axiom of his existence. However, as we will describe, an erotomaniac side to transference demonstrated how Hans did not so much look for love in the Other but answered to the love of the Other. The themes of being 'excluded', 'abandoned', and 'useless' often appeared in the e-mails Hans sent and in the titles of his sculptures; he did not feel like he participated in the social world, and he felt doomed to remain an outsider.

Finally, waves of negative affect were experienced in the body (in the absence of words to reflect on these states): Hans suffered from headaches, nausea, insomnia, and unspecified restlessness. Moreover, he had tinnitus which had preoccupied him for the last two years. He had consulted numerous specialists about his tinnitus, to no avail; no lesions had been found. These bodily experiences emerged unexpectedly, and he was unable to link these sensations to any feeling, thought, or event. Hans noted in one of the first sessions that he had felt nauseous after the previous session. Moreover, even speaking seemed to exacerbate some problematic bodily experiences. These bodily repercussions of his speech, along with the profound inability to express himself and appear as a subject in relation to his life history and his living circumstances further showed the difficulties he had using language as a tool to give meaning to his experiences. We interpret these phenomena as an inability to regulate invasive *jouissance* through the signifier; our hypothesis is that the bodily symptoms reflected an excessive tension that could not be regulated through others and could not be expressed symbolically. Additionally, the overwhelming sadness, the negative affect that appeared out of nowhere (meaning that it is not bound by the signifier or through a history), testified to this incessant resurgence of a dimension of *jouissance*.

Missed encounters and crossing boundaries

In the very first session, Hans gave an account of a series of broken-down relations with mental health professionals. His last psychiatrist told him that he could call her on the phone, but when he did so a few times, he recounts, she told him that he couldn't call her anymore. Following this, he sent her an e-mail, in which he complained about some elements of the treatment; he said she told him that his e-mail had an ungrateful tone and that she really did not like receiving that kind of correspondence. She added that he should have been grateful for the effort she had already put into his treatment, Hans recounts. A previous psychiatric treatment ended with him being hospitalized after he sought out his psychiatrist at her holiday home because she hadn't responded to his phone calls, and he had not heard from her. He talked positively about one psychiatrist, who was humorous, but at the same time confrontational, and treatment with this psychiatrist was terminated because the psychiatrist had to move to another hospital, far away.

Hans was diagnosed by a psychiatrist as having a personality disorder with both dependent and avoidant traits. The problems in the social sphere, which have also manifested with several mental health professionals, were the basis for this diagnosis. Relations with mental health professionals had often ended in a breach with them. From a descriptive point of view, the label of dependent personality disorder seems fit. Interruptions in the treatment due to unforeseen circumstances or holidays were met with great difficulty. It is not uncommon for analysands to suffer from the analyst's absences. However, Hans did not know how to manage these absences.

In my sessions with Hans, the development of transference demonstrated how similar difficulties emerged which made it necessary to develop interventions to counter this pattern. At the end of the first session, Hans asked me to tell him when he goes too far. Although I originally responded that he could say anything he wanted to, I changed my position on this following an incident that occurred after the third session. Hans had phoned me to apologize because he felt he had not been very kind to me, while I had been very friendly to him when showing him out of the door. Hans felt that he didn't respond kindly enough. Even though this was only a minor event that could easily be thought of as an exaggerated form of him wanting to please, I took this incident very seriously for several reasons.

Since Hans concluded the first session by saying that he must be a really difficult person, we could say that this idea now appears in the transferential relationship. Moreover, given how we consider psychotic transference to have the inverted form of neurotic transference, we observed how the perception of love or kindness from the clinician is primary here. I was surprised by Hans's reaction, as I had not expected that being ordinarily courteous would be experienced as anything other than that. Hans, however, felt like he failed to respond to what he had perceived as an act of kindness on my part. From a commonsense perspective, we could assume that being friendly and kind to our patients can facilitate a 'corrective' experience in patients who have experienced a lot of hardships in their relationships with significant others, often from a very early age on. This moment made me aware that the love of the Other could pose difficulties for this patient because it could result in the idea that he is difficult and unresponsive being even more present. Importantly, in these moments he responded to the perception that the Other needed him; when Hans acted upon this need of the Other, he did this as a response to what he perceived to be the Other's intention – an act of love or kindness. This dynamic, however, risked effacing him as a subject, since it reduced him to the object the Other needs, and hence to the *jouissance* of the Other. It became obvious after the intake session that incidents of Hans telephoning mental health professionals and contact outside of the consulting room in general had been critical in the decisions of other health professionals eventually terminating their treatment. The unavailability of one psychiatrist had caused him to cross the line, by looking for her away from the consulting room, during her private time. Importantly, Hans's telephone call to me indicated that he did not interrogate the intention of the Other, but rather jumped to the conclusion that he was at fault.

Waiting ... waiting ... waiting ... in the dark

Hans often talked about situations where others kept him waiting. Their lack of a response posed difficulties because he then felt himself to be at their mercy. The expression he used for this was that he was 'left in the dark'. When someone promised to do something for Hans, he tended to follow a repetitive sequence; he waited and regularly checked whether the person had already fulfilled this promise. If this was not the case, which often occurred, he repeatedly contacted the person to get a response. His tone became demanding and/or disappointed at that point, and if he did not get a response, he called again or sent more e-mails. One report from a previous psychologist mentioned this under the rubric of 'tyrannical' behavior. He stated that Hans was unable to wait and that he expected 'special' treatment. However, this sort of interaction mostly led to Hans feeling bad that he had crossed a line in his communications. He admitted to being angry when others left him waiting. Ambiguous or imprecise messages made him upset and angry: for instance, when he tried to telephone his psychiatrist and got the voicemail message that she was 'unavailable at the moment'. Hans was furious about this because it did not say when she would be back. Interestingly, these communications seemed to ricochet. In the end, he felt like he had gone too far; he insisted too much, or he got carried away by negative feelings, ending up in a position of wordless *jouissance*. Often, an evening of binge drinking – his way of treating *jouissance* – followed, which left him feeling even more like a failure.

This same exchange happened with friends. If a friend canceled an appointment, he would be very upset, but his first reaction was anger or suspicion towards his friend's intentions. Hans thought 'perhaps my friend doesn't want to see me today', but he would always find the ultimate reason for the cancellation in a much deeper conviction of himself being fundamentally unwanted.

He was in psychotherapy with another therapist for over a year and this therapist struggled to contain the disappointment Hans sometimes expressed towards him. Hans wrote him an e-mail in which he complained that the therapist was unavailable. The therapist could only see Hans once a fortnight because this was how the service he worked for was organized; and sometimes he went on holiday without informing Hans well in advance. Moreover, the therapist had promised to call his previous psychiatrist and he had not. The therapist decided to discuss with Hans how this e-mail had affected him *as a person*. He told Hans how much effort he had already put into the therapy and how he felt hurt by the reproaching tone of the e-mail. Hans eventually stopped seeing this therapist because he felt much worse after this type of conversation; he experienced it as if he was the cause of another's suffering: '*It made me feel sick*', he stated. This feeling stuck with him for several days.

Maneuvers in the treatment of the Other

The case of Hans shows how the Other tended to go mad. First, he grappled with an Other that incessantly abandoned him, left him waiting for no obvious reason and was generally disinterested in him. Feeling abandoned obviously does not necessarily point to a manifestation of a psychotic relation to the Other, as it is a common complaint heard in the treatment of (neurotically) depressed patients. However, what is striking is that the abandonment was pervasive and seemed to have a quality of certainty. Whereas a neurotic dynamic is marked by a dialectical interplay with the Other's desire (Does he/she want me? What makes me desirable for the Other?), a psychotic way of relating to the Other always lies at one or other pole of the axis between knowing that the Other wants him (erotomania) and knowing that the Other rejects (paranoia) him. This is the inherent duality in the case of a psychotic structure (Verhaeghe, 2008). Interactions with these faces of the Other, actualized the idea of being worthless and reinforced his belief in being a burden.

The treatment of psychotic subjects is often tackled from the perspective of 'what not to do' (Fink, 2007, p. 234). I aim to unravel my treatment rationale from a more positive perspective, following Lacan's indications on the maneuver of transference. I will describe active interventions that aimed at limiting and regulating excessive *jouissance*, based on the logic of the case.

In search of a limit

One of the most important themes in the treatment was raised by Hans. On concluding the first session, he asked me: 'Will you say when I go too far?'. At first, I responded to this question by inviting him to elaborate, hoping to clarify what these words meant to him. However, when the underlying (psychotic) structure of Hans's suffering became more salient, the clinical strategy changed. As a first important maneuver in the transference, I stated that Hans could not telephone me between sessions. However, he could send me e-mails with what he wanted to say, and he was given reassurance that his e-mails would be discussed in the following session. The underlying motive for this intervention was in the perceived difficulties Hans had managing the absence of the Other, not in the comfort of the analyst[5]. The intervention aimed to prevent the occurrence of moments when Hans would feel the need to cross a boundary ('go too far'), by installing this boundary in the therapeutic frame.

What is more, I stated that I would indicate when Hans had crossed the line or when he went too far. I did so on several occasions: when Hans did call once because he was worried when he drank too much, and when he became insistent and demanding towards other professionals (e.g., his GP) in his communications. These interventions aimed to limit *jouissance* and avoid his actions leading to him feeling bad or suffering from nausea or bodily tension afterward. I didn't explore what the question of "going too far" meant for Hans. I committed myself as a partner in the process of Hans's search for a limit; however, this did not mean that the treatment became directive or restrictive in a general sense. Rather, following Hans's discourse closely, several themes emerged that were central to his feelings of crossing the line.

Free flowing exchanges: interrupting self-hatred

The root of his feeling of having crossed the line is the idea of being a worthless person and the *jouissance* attached to it. In that sense, finding a limit to certain behaviors he felt were transgressive essentially boiled down to finding ways to avoid the idea of being 'a difficult', 'worthless', 'burdensome', ... person, becoming too present. When Hans's discourse became increasingly self-destructive in a session, I interrupted him and actively introduced a different topic; I asked Hans about volunteer work, for instance. As is often the case in melancholia, the *jouissance* of his self-reproach was not canceled out by speaking about it but might rather have been maintained by it (Zenoni, 2008). Being too empathetic at that point would have amounted to being an ally to his most intimate destructiveness. So as to make another discourse possible, it was necessary to regularly halt this type of speech. This conversational style could be characterized as 'free flowing exchanges': different topics could be discussed, one after the other, but without the intention of creating a linear narrative, neither looking for connectedness nor repetition between themes. I actively indicated topics by asking about a range of things that mattered to Hans (e.g., What creative project are you currently working on? How are the dogs? How is your father? What are you reading?); mostly when the self-deprecating thoughts and self-reproach threatened to dominate the session. Speaking in itself did not annul this *jouissance* of self-hatred, so it was necessary to actively put a stop to it.

Communication and alcohol

Hans felt he transgressed social norms, even though he attested to not knowing the rules of communication; he wanted to learn when his communication could be perceived by the other as a reproach. Therefore, his position was akin to the main character in Kafka's novel *The trial*, who is put on the stand but remains in the dark as to the charges made by the prosecution. In the session, I introduced the idea that every communication is essentially flawed; people sometimes hear a message differently than intended. Moreover, I added, that when misunderstandings do occur, this always involves at least two people: no one can be held solely responsible for miscommunication. The idea behind these interventions was to introduce a little space for error in the Other. However, I did not consider the communication *per se* to be the problem. Although undoubtedly Hans struggled with communication, the underlying dynamic had to do with *jouissance* (either of being worthless or being at the mercy of an abandoning Other). By pointing to communication, I attempted to divert the idea that the fault lay on Hans's side alone; others have problems too and communication in itself is distorted.

When Hans felt he had transgressed or when he felt excessively bad or worthless, he took recourse to alcohol. After having a lot to drink, he felt he had gone too far. The drinking can be seen as a form of self-medication, an attempt at regulating *jouissance* that bypasses the Other – when too many bad things had come out of his mouth, he put bad things in it (alcohol). Afterwards, the guilt over having drank too much (again) pervaded him. In the sessions, I proposed that he drank less because of its aftereffects, by asking for instance, 'What else could you do when you feel bad?'

Time

Lacanian therapists demonstrate flexibility regarding how they use frequency and time, standard elements of the analytic situation or frame, to have interpretative effects in analyses with neurotic subjects. In psychosis, however, time is not used to make particular themes or signifiers resonate in between sessions. Following the logic in Hans's case particularly, the framework was tailored to a standard weekly session of 50 minutes. Variable sessions could put too much emphasis on the arbitrariness of the analyst; they risk putting the analyst in the place of an almighty and whimsical Other. Time is a symbolic aspect of life[6] that has an important role both in the experience of psychosis as well as in the handling of the therapeutic frame. Of course, time also regulates a lot of social practices in general. It is one of the signatures of modern times, that we live by the clock. If the analyst adheres to a fixed time, this conveys how he is a dupe of a symbolic pact as well – the analyst is not a character out of time but someone who suffers the same time limit as anyone else. The framework of the therapy thus constituted a ritualized practice. However, whereas in neurotic subjects this would risk alienating the patient and eventually lead to a stagnation in the therapy, this ritualization constitutes the creation of a mini version of the social bond. Moreover, the ritual counters the duality and the attribution of meaning to the therapist's interventions – meaning becomes deflated, because the Other has a certain predictability, leaving less room for interpretations of malevolence.

Interpreter of the mad Other

Given that, for Hans, the Other is mad, treatment should be aimed at this Other. In the case of Hans, it is remarkable how the Other seemed to appear without a clear rationale. There was something opaque and undecipherable to the Other, which left him at the mercy of the Other's whims. In that sense, the most important pitfall to avoid was becoming another incarnation of an abandoning and uninterpretable Other. One of the ways to achieve this was through interpreting myself as a therapist so that my interventions and behaviors were framed and understandable. This could be done by reference to how clinicians adhering to my psychoanalytic school of thought behave and act in a therapeutic session, which was intended to convey the message to Hans that he was not at the mercy of my personal whims but that I also had rules to adhere to. For instance, once he said he found it extremely difficult that he could not call me in between sessions; I responded that in psychoanalytic therapy in general, the work is done in sessions. Another way of achieving this was through small self-disclosures. For example, after one session he e-mailed me because he was upset by my repeatedly yawning during the last session; in the next session, I told him that I had indeed been very sleepy because I had been woken up several times during the night. This was indeed the case, but more importantly, it conveyed how my behavior had a cause outside of the therapeutic relationship. I do not believe that this type of intervention works because it is authentic or congruent (Rogers 1957), but rather because it makes little cracks in the all too present *jouissance* of the Other. Note that this type of intervention is different from the actions of Hans' last therapist: I did not pinpoint Hans's behavior or communication as a cause for my feelings or behavior.

Similarly, one of the ways in which extra-transferential difficulties with others were handled was through interpreting the behavior of these others differently than as an indication that the Other was committed to him completely. Then, Hans and I looked for the rules that governed the Other's behavior. Sometimes, I took recourse to more general theories on communication, explaining how there is necessarily an aspect of distortion of the intended message to it. Moreover, when Hans recounted feuds with relatives or friends, I focused on alternative explanations for their behavior. I proposed some hypotheses about why someone would have responded in a short fashion, or not at all – maybe they had a bad day or maybe they did not quite know how to respond to his communication? This operation of castrating the Other, aims at countering a too massive and committed Other and trying to decipher the enigma that the Other presents.

Working with Hans's affinities

In line with a psychoanalytic approach to the treatment of autism (Maleval & Grollier, 2017), my work with Hans consisted of working with his affinities. In the past, Hans had sometimes come across others who were helpful to him; he had good experiences during his time in residential settings. When exploring these experiences, he mentioned that they showed an interest in him, and stimulated him; it was a safe environment and he felt accepted for who he was.[7] The exploration of this experience, indicated that showing an interest in *what he does,* rather than what he *is*, had a positive impact on his wellbeing. I did show interest and actively questioned him, inviting him to elaborate on certain practices that helped him to limit his sadness and even find some pleasure from time to time. I asked Hans repeatedly about what he was sculpting: What was his project? What material would he use? What composition? What subject did he want to express? Importantly, when he brought pictures of his work, sketches, or drawings, I did not extensively probe into matters such as the meaning of the work, the real subject, or what might be hidden under the surface. Rather, Hans was invited to talk about the process of constructing the work, how he went about it, what he would do with it, the colors, the composition, and the material.

Hans was 'looking for something to hold on to'. He had tried several activities in the past, with this aim. Hans read a lot, wrote, sculpted, and worked as a volunteer at an animal shelter; I actively stimulated him to turn to these activities when feeling bad.

Discussion

The case of Hans demonstrates the many faces of transference (Nobus, 2000) in a case of psychosis. In relation to his previous psychiatrist and psychologist, the dynamic became one of erotomaniac transference wherein Hans was the object of the Other's love. The phone call where he apologized for not being kind enough revealed how the love of the Other needs to be addressed by him: the Other's initiative and love were primary. According to Zenoni (2008), in psychosis, transference has an inverse structure: from the Other to the subject – here, Hans was the object of the *jouissance* of the Other, both in terms of love as well as hate (where a more paranoid coloring infiltrated his experience of the Other). Prior treatments fell prey to the pitfalls of this dual transferential relationship, and, in my work with Hans, I attempted to avoid this position. In order to maintain a manageable transference, I described how I tried to counter this position of the Other in the treatment by signifying a limit. Moreover, both myself, as well as others, were interpreted, so as to put a limit to my own and their whimsicality. However, I did not interpret or explain the relation I had to Hans. The relation to the Other was to a large extent the focus of the treatment, studying and interpreting this in order for Hans to find a position where he was not the object of the Other. This meant a perpetual translation of the enigmatic Other to avoid ending up in the position of being prey to the Other's *jouissance*. Even though Hans's relation to the Other was a central topic in the treatment, it was never interpreted from the here and now of the therapeutic relationship. Rather, I tried to continuously open up a space where Hans could create solutions for himself.

What became more prominent as treatment progressed, was the way the case was centered around a relation of intimacy and *jouissance* with the object *a* (melancholia). Hans *was* the disposable object. Most of his speech revolved around how he feels he is a worthless burden. His position of exclusion was also evident in the poetry he wrote, where the impossibility of finding a place in the social world was one of the most important themes. Nevertheless, he continued his attempts to establish a link or a connection with the Other, but ultimately, he was recast to his position as an object – this corroborates with the complexity of the case. When Hans tried to connect to the Other, he encountered the Other's *jouissance*. However, ultimately, this fell back on him, and the end result was a reinforcement of the ideas of nullity that he so intimately entertains. In that sense, both his relation to the self, as well as his relation to the Other, were consistent with the self-reproaches. He encountered the position of being an outcast time and again, even though he kept trying to enter the social circuit. Ultimately, his interests allowed him to occupy some positions (e.g., volunteer work) that gave him an identity, a structure to his week, and a position among others where he could feel safe and valuable. An important part of the treatment was made up of supporting these solutions.

The case study exemplifies how transference had both an erotomaniacal, as well as a more solipsistic side (self-loathing) in this case, thus requiring a multitude of maneuvers of transference. These *maneuvers* are interventions aimed at countering an invasive *jouissance* through the analytic frame, naming certain aspects of experience and framing the Other. Besides the position of the clinician, this also has implications for the aim of the treatment. Leader (2011) points to the importance of endurance in this type of clinical work. Even though some psychotic subjects succeed in inventing a practice that helps regulate *jouissance* in a few sessions, Hans's case demonstrated a treatment process that was more supportive in nature; Hans was pervaded by a sense of hopelessness and reproached himself for not being able to change: 'I have been in psychotherapy for so long and still I feel this sadness'. At one point during the treatment, Hans brought a letter that he wrote during his stay in the hospital over 10 years ago. The content of the letter was very similar to a lot of the content of the sessions and the things he had been expressing in the treatment thus far. He noticed this himself, which came as somewhat of a shock to him: 'nothing has changed'. He seemed to be caught up in an eternity of suffering. Indeed, in Hans's case and in the case of melancholia in general, the aim of treatment is not to get rid of the negative effect so as to get on with life, but through treatment to try to find a way for the analysand to be able to cope with people and experiences, in general, going forward. A highly intensive focus on therapeutic effects would risk backfiring because he would have been confronted even more with difficulties that persist. However, one of the (explicit) aims of the treatment was to try to find a way, through clinical dialogue, that Hans could cope with his social environment and with social interactions that debilitated him. Additionally, the clinician looked for ways in which the overwhelming feelings could be channeled and for Hans to be able to experience joy, excitement, and pleasure in general. This was approached through supporting his projects, not by analyzing his personality or the transference.

Notes

1 Miller (1999) distinguishes between what he calls 'six paradigms of *jouissance*' in Lacan's oeuvre, each reflecting a different understanding of the relation between language and *jouissance*.
2 The French adjective 'mortifiant' means: offensive, humiliating, mortifying, injuring, insulting, harming self-love.
3 In the English translation of the Écrits by Bruce Fink 'manoeuvre du transfert' is translated as 'handling of transference'. We choose to use our own translation that remains closer to the French with its connotative implication of a necessary movement on the side of the analyst.
4 In the Lacanian movement this is called 'ordinary psychosis' (see Redmond, 2013).
5 This is not a one-size-fits-all intervention. For some patients it can be wise to maintain a certain accessibility, even when on vacation or during the holidays. The clinical decision on how to manage this, should (ideally) be motivated by the logic of the case, not the possible countertransferential experience of the clinician (for instance, feeling worried about or suffocated by a patient).
6 An extensive body of literature exists on the relation between time and psychoanalysis. For a Lacanian interpretation of this topic, we refer the reader to Johnston (2005).
7 We could assume that one of the reasons why the residential setting was a good place for him, was in the fact that transference was distributed among several persons (the nurses, psychiatrist, creative therapists and other members of the staff). Typically, work with psychotic subjects is distributed among several people, so as to divide up transference, making it less immense.

References

Cauwe, J., Vanheule, S. & Desmet, M. (2017) 'The Presence of the Analyst in Lacanian Treatment', *Journal of the American Psychoanalytic Association*, 65, pp. 609–638.
Facchin, F. (2016) 'Psychoses without Symptoms and Stabilized Psychoses: Lacanian Suggestions for Treating Fuzzy Contemporary Clinical Phenomena', *British Journal of Psychotherapy*, 32, pp. 21–36.
Fink, B. (2007) *Fundamental of Psychoanalytic Technique. A Lacanian Approach for Practitioners*. New York: Norton.
Freud, S. (1914) 'On Narcissism: An Introduction', in J. Strachey (Ed.), *The Standard Edition of the Complete Psychological Works of Sigmund Freud*, Volume 14. London: The Hogarth Press and the Institute of Psycho-Analysis, pp. 161–215.

Freud, S. (1917) 'Mourning and Melancholia', in J. Strachey (Ed.), *The Standard Edition of the Complete Psychological Works of Sigmund Freud*, Volume 14. London: The Hogarth Press and the Institute of Psycho-Analysis, pp. 237–58.

Grigg, R. (2015) 'Melancholia and the Unabandoned Object', in P. Gherovici & M. Steinkoler (eds), *Lacan on Madness. Madness, Yes You Can't*. London and New York: Routledge, pp. 139–158.

Johnston, A. (2005) *Time Driven: Metapsychology and the Splitting of the Drive*. Evanston: Northwestern University Press.

Lacan, J. (1951) 'Presentation on Transference', in B. Fink (trans.), *Écrits*. New York: Norton, pp. 176–185.

Lacan, J. (1959) 'On a Question Prior to Any Possible Treatment of Psychosis', in B. Fink (trans.), *Écrits*. New York: Norton, pp. 445–488.

Lacan, J. (1960–61) *Le Séminaire. Livre VIII: Le Transfert*, ed. J.-A. Miller. Paris: Seuil.

Lacan, J. (1966) 'Présentation des Mémoires d'un Névropathe', in J.-A. Miller (ed.), *Autres Écrits*. Paris: Seuil, pp. 213–218.

Lacan, J. (2014) *The Seminar. Book X: Anxiety (1963–1963)*, trans. A.R. Price, ed, J.-A. Miller. Cambridge: Polity Press.

Leader, D. (2008) *The New Black. Mourning, Melancholia and Depression*. London: Penguin Books.

Leader, D. (2011) *What Is Madness?* London: Hamish Hamilton.

Maleval, J.-C. (2015) 'Treatment of the Psychoses and Contemporary Psychoanalysis', in P. Gherovici & M. Steinkoler (eds.), *Lacan on Madness: Madness, Yes You Can't*. London and New York: Routledge, pp. 99–111.

Maleval, J.-C. & Grollier, M. (2017) 'La Thérapie par Affinités (ou le Résistible Retour d'une Approche Psychodynamique pour le Traitement des Autistes) [Affinity Therapy (or the Resistible Return of a Psychodynamic Approach for the Treatment of Autism)]', *L'évolution psychiatrique* 82, pp. 646–663.

Miller, J.-A. (1999) 'Paradigms of Jouissance', *Lacanian Ink*, 17, pp. 8–47.

Nobus, D. (2000) *Jacques Lacan and the Freudian Practice of Psychoanalysis*. New York: Routledge.

Redmond, J. (2013) 'Contemporary Perspectives on Lacanian Theories of Psychosis', *Frontiers in Psychology*, 4, pp. 350, 1–15.

Rogers, C. R. (1957) 'The Necessary and Sufficient Conditions of Therapeutic Personality Change', *Journal of Consulting Psychology*, 21, pp. 97–103.

Vanheule, S. (2011) *The Subject of Psychosis: A Lacanian Perspective*. London and New York: Palgrave Macmillan.

Verhaeghe, P. (2008) *On Being Normal and Other Disorders. A Manual for Clinical Psychodiagnostics*, trans. S. Jottkandt. London: Karnac Books.

Zenoni, A. (2008) 'De Logica van de Overdracht in de Psychose [The Logic of Transference in Psychosis]', *iNWiT*, 13, pp. 139–163.

Chapter 7

The complex of melancholia

Derek Hook

The aim of this chapter is to explore key facets of melancholia by referring both to a clinical case and to the tragic story of Christopher McCandless as retold in Jon Krakauer's (1996) *Into the Wild*, Sean Penn's (2007) film of the same name, and his sister, Carine McCandless's story (2014) *The Wild Truth*. My more specific aims are twofold. First, I want to engender a distinctively Lacanian perspective on melancholia. Second, bearing in mind Freud's (1923) remark that in melancholia we observe "a pure culture of the death instinct" (p. 53), I want to foreground the role of the death drive in melancholia. As will soon become apparent, the approach I will develop toward melancholia may initially appear at odds with Freud's (1917) account which focuses largely on the role of a previously loved yet subsequently hated and internalized lost object. A different set of conceptual priorities comes to the fore in a Lacanian reading, particularly so given Lacan's insistence on the death drive as enacted *within* the symbolic realm. This is the death drive understood not as a quasi-biological or organic force, nor as most fundamentally a will to self-annihilation. The Lacanian death drive is instead a type of *life in excess of life*, and it entails the wish to break from – even destroy – the network of given symbolic roles, debts, and obligations that structure social existence.

I am not the first to stress a series of Lacanian postulates regarding melancholia that differs from Freudian conceptualizations (Leader, 2003, 2008). I begin this chapter by citing Russell Grigg's (2015) recent argument that it is the *presence* of the object rather than its absence that is most crucial in melancholia. Building on this challenge to Freud's conceptualization, I sketch a brief outline of a clinical case and then turn to the story of Christopher McCandless (Krakauer, 1996; McCandless, 2014; Penn, 2007). After elaborating upon a striking series of similarities between these two cases, I conclude by stressing a series of ideas relating to the death drive in melancholia that a Lacanian frame of reference allows us to foreground.

The over-proximity of the object

Even those with only a passing familiarity with Freud's (1917) *Mourning and Melancholia* are acquainted with the idea that the melancholic suffers from the

DOI: 10.4324/9781003216391-8

loss of a once loved and then subsequently hated object. Following this account, the melancholic, having narcissistically identified with the object, wages a clamorous psychical war against it *via the medium of their own ego*. We are thus able to explain one of the key features of melancholia repeatedly stressed by Freud (1917), namely the fact that the constant complaints and allegations that the melancholic directs against themselves sound very much as if they fit another object altogether.

While we should not of course jettison Freud's account, it is worthwhile interrogating whether it is the *loss* of an object that plays the predominant role. Put differently, we might ask whether the loss of an *imaginary* (ego-supporting) object may not be coterminous with the invasive presence of an object of a different order – that of the Lacanian *real* – which cannot be kept at bay. This argument is advanced by Grigg (2015) who observes, in respect of psychoanalytic transference that "it is the very presence of the object, rather than its loss, that is critical [in melancholia]" (p. 152). "[M]elancholia", as such "is not about object loss"; "mourning ... which is produced by the loss of an object, is a misleading model for melancholia" (p. 152).

A crucial facet of Grigg's disagreement with Freud is the idea that the attack upon the self in melancholia is too devastating to be understood as internalized aggression against the object. One might retort here that Grigg is not giving the sadistic and punitive agency of the superego the prominence it deserves in the dynamics of melancholia. (Grigg is somewhat dismissive when it comes to affording the superego an explanatory role in melancholia). Nevertheless, he has an important point: the damage experienced by the subject, the eruption of harmful *jouissance* – indeed, the toxicity of the object – seems to exceed what can be accounted for in terms of superego violence.

Let us turn directly to Grigg's account:

> What makes melancholia so different from mourning is that the melancholic subject turns out to be defenceless against the object. The object cannot be memorialized, as in mourning, and instead remains forever there in the real. The collapse of semblants that otherwise veil the object persists, and the "grimace" of the object, like the grimace of a skull behind a beautiful face, is exposed; for the melancholic, the veil of semblants, the *i(a)* over the object *a* falls altogether.
>
> (p. 153)

Crucial here is the distinction between *imaginary* or ego-sustaining objects (*semblants*) which provide a type of fantasy covering, and the *real* object which occurs minus any protective screen. This object – which Grigg equates with Lacan's object *a* – is not merely the object-cause of desire, as it is so often characterized in secondary literature. In its real, which is to say its *unmediated* and 'unprocessable' form, this 'object' is also traumatic – an excessive thing that promises to irradiate the subject with inflammatory *jouissance*. This unscreened object exerts a type of toxic over-proximity, an over-proximity which means that

> the subject has not separated himself from it as [...] object cause of desire. This separation, which for the neurotic subject is produced by the Other as locus of speech and language, both regulates and limits his *jouissance*. In the absence of this separation a plenitude of *jouissance* is apparent in such [...] formations as erotomania, hypochondriasis, and the persecutions characteristic of paranoia. [...] In melancholia we encounter the same failure of separation from the object. The depressive function is explained by the fact that the unseparated-off object, in being a "piece of the real" [...] leaves the subject exposed and defenceless to its ravages.
>
> (p. 154)

I am perhaps more persuaded than Grigg that such an over-proximity of the real object can be read as compatible with the basic outline of Freud's (1917) model of melancholia. Nevertheless, one appreciates what motivates his account. Firstly, he wants to underline a more radical distinction between mourning and melancholia than he sees in Freud's description (and here one must agree: mourning is in no way an adequate paradigm within which to broach the nature of melancholia). Furthermore, Grigg wishes to stress the severity, indeed, the *psychotic* nature of melancholia, which becomes evident precisely given the vulnerability of the psychotic subject before the toxic object.

It helps here to stress that the neurotic subject has the resources of fantasy and desire, recourse to an Other (of language, of prevailing socio-symbolic norms and values) to help absorb such a traumatic impact. In this respect, the Other is a point of appeal, a place to which one can direct one's complaints or objections. Similarly, the Other as a site of shared social meaning can provide a symbolic frame, a means of speaking about and thereby diffusing anxieties and harmful *jouissance*; this Other can be used as a resource for narrativization. Such *jouissance*-management strategies are not as available to the psychotic subject who, to risk a broad structural generalization, lacks the buffers to *jouissance* mobilized by the neurotic.

Seceding from the symbolic: A case summary

One of the challenges of psychoanalysis as a 'science of the particular' (Verhaeghe, 2001) lies in grasping how a highly distinctive set of symptoms is also 'universal', at least in the sense of belonging to a broad diagnostic structure. Something of this challenge was apparent in the case of a patient I worked with some years ago, who presented with a series of puzzling symptoms, some of which seemed, on the face of it, to have little or nothing to do with melancholia. Several key themes came to the fore in the clinical work, which I list, schematically, below.

1. **Difficulties in receiving gifts/symbolic marking:** The patient experienced extreme difficulty – and a considerable degree of anxiety – in situations where he was forced to receive gifts. Such an aversive reaction was apparent not just in the case of gifts from family and friends, but even when he was given small tokens of gratitude from work colleagues. To receive any token of the Other's desire was, in short, a painfully excessive experience. Even as a child he disliked receiving gifts, and he frequently contrived to get his birthday forgotten. One way he devised of dealing with this difficulty was to transfer such gifts. This was an effective way of enacting a reversal from the position of a recipient to a giving position.

   In one particular case, the effects of receiving a large gift proved disastrous: it brought a longstanding intimate relationship to an unhappy end. This problem with accepting gifts was evident also in my patient's disinclination to accept any remuneration offered by his place of work beyond his usual salary. His preference for *giving to* (rather than receiving from) others was also apparent in a long-held wish to work for a charity. Related to this was his profound distaste for what he considered to be the unethical business practices of large financial institutions. He wished, by contrast, to play a part in redistributing rather than accumulating wealth. His preoccupations with avoiding gifts and charitable giving often took on a severe super-ego quality.

   My working theory was that he disliked his existence being too forcefully acknowledged *or symbolically marked* by any desiring Other. Much by the same token, he avoided, wherever possible, being locked into reciprocal relations of exchange that fixed him in a designated symbolic role. His interest in charity seemed to fit this idea: his aversion to receiving gifts seemed largely to be about avoiding indebtedness, avoiding being locked into a relationship of obligation, which itself indicates how one is tied into a symbolic place that one detests or simply feels unable to maintain.

2. **An inability to mediate intimacy (the 'terror of closeness'):** My patient also experienced great difficulties in managing personal relationships. Romantic relationships would invariably become too intense and he struggled to strike the right distance between the extremes of aloofness and suffocating proximity. This occurred in both social and more intimate relationships. There seemed to be no happy medium, no balance between his powerful need for distance from social others and the occasional bout of uninhibited and ultimately damaging intimacy. Just as he experienced a 'terror' of gifts, so he exhibited what Verhaeghe (2004) refers to as a 'terror of closeness'. He knew no viable way of moderating intimacy, of introducing a screen between himself and the Other.

   An accomplished sailor and solo yachtsman, my patient managed his problem of intimacy by participating in an exhausting – and often dangerous – series of regattas and one-man sailing events all across the United States. For a lengthy period, participation in such events provided a solitary escape from intimate relations and social obligations alike; virtually all of his time was spent training for, traveling to or participating in such events. This difficulty in mediating relationships chimes with Grigg's (2015) description of the over-proximity of the object in melancholia and his related suggestion that such an "unseparated off" object exerts a type of unscreened *jouissance*.

3. **A yearning for anonymity and disappearance:** My patient had a frequent need to uproot himself, to cut social and professional ties, to move from one job or residential address to another. He periodically abandoned email accounts and cell numbers, starting afresh with new contact details that he shared with as few people as possible. Being in any one position for too long elicited considerable anxiety; long-term recognizability was almost unbearable for him. He felt acutely the weight of social relationships with people whom he was certain he would, in due course, disappoint. He experienced his existence as unworthy, undeserved, as – and here we are more clearly within the realm of melancholia – blameworthy and a reason for guilt. His negative self-evaluations invoked Freud's description according to which the melancholic patient "describes his ego [...] as being worthless [...] morally reprehensible, he is filled with self-reproach, he levels insults against himself and exerts ostracism and punishment" (Freud, 1917, p. 313).

This certainty that others would soon discover his worthlessness was perhaps why he so frequently voiced the wish to become anonymous, to bypass any forms of symbolic registration – permanent roles, positions, relationships, etc. The reverie that he often experienced when talking of his more grueling sailing events was one of disappearance or demise, of going 'off grid', being lost and never found. He had broken off all relations with his parents and extended family years ago, and he maintained an unconditional hatred for his father.

4. **Existing in a twilight world:** The patient's day-to-day thoughts were punctuated with images of his suicide. He had a richly developed and well-researched set of ideas about how this might be most effectively accomplished. Additionally, he often described what I thought of as 'twilight scenes', scenarios in which he, or others, were suspended between the worlds of the living and dead. Typically, these were scenarios in which people were poised on the threshold of their death or were surrounded by those who had already passed into another world. These images conveyed something of his everyday experience. He existed in a state preoccupied with death, a condition that was incommensurable with the world of the living, and near impossible to explain to those around him. This condition of opting out of social life, while at the same time endlessly contemplating actual suicide – the state of being *between two deaths* in Lacan's (1992) memorable phrase – is ultimately what made life bearable for him. Leader's (2008) description of the melancholic's existence as split between "the 'unreal' world of social being" (p. 182) on the one hand, and their 'real' existence, of "absolute solitude" (p. 174), on the other hand, that proves particularly poignant here. The same is true of Verhaeghe's (2004)

comment that, in melancholia, "the subject is empty, has nothing ... is a member of the living dead ... [who] takes the entire guilt of the world onto its shoulders" (p. 455).

It took me a while to understand that my patient's twilight scenes and his associated reveries of suicide were not indications of imminent risk. They served instead a consoling function; the painful condition of his existence was assuaged rather than exacerbated through such imaginings. His melancholia was not simply about a drive to suicide; it was a more complex negotiation whereby the presence of (imaginary and symbolic) death enabled him to live. Perhaps the most telling example of his melancholic state was his wish not merely to die, but that his life would be somehow retrospectively erased, such that he had never lived at all. This desire for complete erasure was apparent in an obstacle he ran up against when contemplating suicide. He had the discomforting thought that there would inevitably be some remainder – his body, traces of the suicidal act – which someone would discover, and which would call attention both to the fact that he had lived and to the relationships which had in some respect defined him.[1] Of course, this was precisely the opposite of what he wanted, which was to disappear quite literally without a trace, without affirming the fact of his symbolic existence, without revitalizing the historical social and familial relationships that he so desperately wanted to erase.

Disturbances in the symbolic

If we are to bring a Lacanian perspective to this case material, two features, in particular, are worth stressing. Firstly – following Grigg (2015) – melancholia can be approached not only – or even chiefly – as the problem of a once loved now lost object. Melancholia can just as well be conceptualized as a difficulty with being definitively located, *marked* in the symbolic. This may be apparent in family/social relations as the melancholic experiences are unbearable and claustrophobic. It may likewise be apparent in a reticence to receive gifts or any tokens of the Other's desire that locates the subject within a series of obligations. This difficulty is thus the flip side of the problem with mediating intimacy ('the terror of closeness'), in which relations with the Other seem either to plunge into suffocating over-proximity or to fall apart altogether. The question of an optimal distance to the Other, who is somehow excessive, of course, resonates with Grigg's description of the 'too muchness' of object a. The object a in this respect is the traumatic kernel, the 'little piece of the Real' which, like the skull beneath the face that Grigg so memorably invokes, shines through the Other to exert its traumatic influence on the melancholic subject.

So, whereas Grigg, following a reading of the later Lacan, emphasizes the over-proximity of object a, I have stressed difficulties in the allocation of a symbolic role, what we might call a crisis of marking. Of course, from a Lacanian perspective – a point worth stressing – *these are two sides of the same coin.* Difficulties in taking up a stable position relative to the desire of the Other are, at once, problems of symbolic placement *and* of the failure to regulate the damaging *jouissance* emitting from the object *a* in the Other. In other words, it is not just the symbolic relation to the Other that is the problem. There is also a crisis concerning what is in the Other (what 'in them is more than them'), the dilemma of the object *a* within the Other that has come too close.[2] And it has come too close precisely because the melancholic subject lacks the means of symbolic mediation necessary to protect themselves from it.

Life beyond life

While not obviously present in the first sections of the foregoing case summary, the death drive is clearly enough in evidence in the last of the themes discussed. The extreme maritime risks and challenges that my patient undertook every week took him 'beyond the pleasure principle', far exceeding what could, in any ordinary terms of reference, be considered to be either healthy or enjoyable. We should nonetheless add a clarifying proviso here, pointing out that the death drive, for Lacan, is apparent less in a literal wish to die, than in a type of *life in excess of life.* The death drive, following this tack, is apparent in activities of surplus vitality, in forms of unnatural ('undead') libidinal animation (*jouissance*) that override the biological imperatives of adaptation and self-preservation. It is for this reason that Lacan insists that the death drive is not "a perversion of instinct but rather a desperate affirmation of life" (1992, p. 263). As Žižek puts it:

> The Freudian death drive has nothing whatsoever to do with the craving for self-annihilation [...] it is, on the contrary, the very opposite of dying – a name for the "undead" eternal life itself [...] The paradox of the Freudian "death drive" is therefore that it is Freud's name for its very opposite, for the way immortality appears within psychoanalysis, for an uncanny excess of life, for an 'undead' urge which persists beyond the (biological) cycle of life and death [...] The ultimate lesson of psychoanalysis is that human life is never 'just life': humans are not simply alive, they are possessed by the strange drive to enjoy life in excess, passionately attached to a surplus which sticks out and derails the ordinary run of things.
>
> (Žižek, 2006, p. 61)

We might differ slightly from Žižek here, since the death drive might indeed – as in the current case – be signaled by a craving for self-annihilation, even if this is not its only or even its most salient feature. However, Žižek's remarks remain instructive since they overturn the assumption that melancholia should be understood along the lines of a severe and/or encompassing mode of depression, and withdrawal. The death drive doubtless appears also in moments of 'unholy' stimulation, in *jouissance*-inducing highs, in the libidinal gratifications of the transgressive or the extreme. It is in such moments that the experience of being most fully alive comes full circle to embrace the limits or excesses of life more typically associated with death.

Into the Wild

Christopher McCandless grew up in an upper-middle-class Washington DC suburb, graduating, with honors, from Emory University in 1990. After graduating, McCandless donated his life savings ($24,000.00) to charity, abandoned his car and the majority of his possessions, gave up his birth name (more on this later), and went off-grid. Adopting the life of a wanderer, he moved across the United States, picking up jobs here and there, living the solitary existence of a free spirit beholden to no one. He could not be traced or reached by his family, who had lost any sense of where he might be until his body was discovered by hikers in Alaska.

McCandless's death in rural Alaska – suffering from hunger, he had misidentified a harmful plant as edible, eaten it, and died as a result – captured the public's imagination when it occurred. A brief overview of McCandless's story will allow us to highlight a series of components that bear a striking resemblance to the case discussed above. My intention here is neither to 'pathologize' McCandless nor to provide a type of retrospective diagnosis. Given that I am familiar with McCandless only through the existing literature, any attempt at the latter would be ill-advised. That being said, there do seem to be several extraordinary parallels between these cases and exploring them might assist us in grasping a series of clinical motifs typical of melancholia. A point of clinical diagnostics should be stressed here. That a biographical account may contain symptomatic features illustrative of a diagnostic structure *does not* mean that the individual in question should necessarily be diagnosed as such. This gap between apparent symptoms and diagnostic structure should be borne in mind as we consider the details of McCandless's story which, to be sure, serves us as a literary reference-point, rather than a clinical instantiation of melancholia.

I noted in my case summary that the melancholic patient I worked with was exceedingly uncomfortable in situations in which he was made to receive gifts; that he preferred to transfer such gifts to others; that charity, rather than the accumulation of wealth, was important to him. I noted also that he disliked being symbolically marked; that he frequently broke off existing social and professional ties when they became either too intimate or threatened to tie him to a given symbolic identity; and that he yearned for anonymity, to disappear without a trace. All of these themes are, in varying ways, apparent in Krakauer's depiction of McCandless.

A considerable portion of the pathos of *Into the Wild* concerns the degree to which McCandless was willing to cut himself off both from his family and from the values and symbolic roles expected of him, to forge instead an entirely different and more solitary life. However, his avoidance of everyday social norms, roles, and obligations had begun some time before he set out on his wilderness adventures. We know that during his early years in Washington DC, McCandless would seek out poverty-stricken areas of the city, striking up conversations with destitute folks and sex workers, sometimes offering to buy them food. We know also that he viewed wealth as corrupting, as a moral vice; he increasingly gravitated to the frugal lifestyle of renunciation and scarcity not so far removed from the living conditions of the poor people he had met in the ghettos of the city. The Russian novelist Tolstoy – the exemplar of an ascetic, self-disciplined, abstentious life – became a role model of sorts, someone McCandless strove to emulate.

A crucial turning point in Sean Penn's (2007) film version of *Into the Wild* – a moment similarly emphasized in Carine McCandless's account of events (2014) – concerns her brother's angry refusal to accept a new car that his parents wanted to give him as a graduation present. In Krakauer's (1996) telling, this refusal – which included also his parents' offer to pay for his studies – took on the force of a moral principle associated with a declared intent not to accept any gifts from them in the future. McCandless planned to blindside his parents, to make a definitive break – indeed, to 'divorce' them – after they had assumed he had come around to their way of thinking. He resolved to cut them out of his life. It is interesting that in both the Christopher McCandless story and the case discussed above, an unwanted gift – which is also of course an unwanted intimacy, an unwanted debt, a 'too muchness' of the Other – featured as a point of rupture. Clearly, like my patient, McCandless evinced a volatile reaction to being the recipient of a gift that would lock him into a designated role (the son of his parents).

Several further incidents can be cited in which Christopher McCandless was either notably uncomfortable with, or attempted his best to sidestep, forms of symbolic marking. An example is a new name McCandless adopted when he began his travels: Alexander Supertramp. Upon reflection, this was not so much a *new* name as the *avoidance* of a name. I say this for two reasons: First, 'Supertramp' seems more a description than a name – McCandless had, after all, embraced the life of a destitute wanderer, albeit of a 'super' (youthful, adventurous) sort. Second, by taking on this particular moniker, McCandless was substituting a well-worn signifier from American popular and literary culture for his name. ('Supertramp' is the name for a famous rock band, and – perhaps more significantly for McCandless – it featured in the title of WH Davies's (1908) book: *The Autobiography of a Super-tramp*[3]). Interestingly, a similar gesture is apparent in the case of another young man Krakauer discusses in *Into the Wild,* the explorer Everett Ruess, who, Krakauer felt, clearly exhibited similar tendencies to McCandless. Ruess sought escape from society in the American wilderness, and ultimately died as a result. He had adopted the name Nemo, the name of the sea captain in Jules Verne's *Twenty Thousand Leagues Under the Sea*. Nemo, of course, also means 'no one' and, as such, it functions in much the same way as does 'Supertramp' – not so much as a name, but as a kind of refuge in anonymity.

The second key theme of the foregoing case study – my patient's difficulty in managing intimate relationships and a sense of feeling suffocated by them – may not immediately seem to fit with what we know of McCandless. McCandless, as portrayed in both the book and film versions of *Into the Wild*, did forge several significant, if short-lived, relationships. There seems little doubt that McCandless could be personable and warm, that many of the people he met were drawn to him. That he could be generous and responsive to others is not in question. However, the prospect of establishing an ongoing intimate relationship with McCandless represented an altogether different proposition. A nice detail in Penn's (2006) film – which closely follows Krakauer's (1996) account – helps put McCandless's apparent sociability into perspective. We see how Ron Franz, a disconsolate old man who had lost his family under tragic circumstances, befriended McCandless and subsequently asked if he might formally adopt him. If my hypothesis regards the aversive reaction (the 'terror of closeness') that McCandless experienced when forced to assume an intimate symbolic bond is correct, then, such an offer was, unbeknownst to Franz, a guaranteed means of pushing McCandless away. McCandless, Krakauer intuits, was uncomfortable with the request, and dodged the question by promising to reconsider it after his Alaskan adventure. Then, relieved to be free from the burden of personal relations and the associated complications of intimacy and its various commitments, McCandless took to the road.

A series of themes come together here: an apparent inability to take a permanent position within an inter-subjective relationship; the need – via forms of anonymity and disappearance – to escape society and bypass symbolic debts and obligations; and the over-proximity of the object, that is, the over-intensity of intimacies that prove impossible to mediate. I barely need to add that all of these considerations can be understood as difficulties *in assuming a symbolic location*. The Lacanian insight is that precisely such difficulties might be considered possible indicators of melancholic structure.

Rather than approaching the McCandless story in the romantic terms of a lone spirit breaking out of a meaningless life, we might pause to consider a different narrative. It may perhaps have been for McCandless, as it was for my patient, that he found the symbolic and social constraints of an everyday existence intolerable, hopelessly difficult to manage. Carine McCandless (2014) implies as much when she insists that, rather than a selfish or irresponsible act, walking into the wild was perhaps the sanest thing her brother could have done. A note that McCandless committed to his journal on February 3, 1991, seems to further corroborate the perspective I am developing. Writing in the third person, McCandless recorded that Alex [Supertramp] went to Los Angeles to find a job, but had become extremely uncomfortable in society, and needed, as such, to return to the road immediately (see Krakauer, 1996, p. 37).[4]

We should also consider an example that may initially appear to refute my argument about McCandless's apparent avoidance of symbolic marking. I have in mind an instance where McCandless gave a gift to his friend and former employer, Wayne Westerberg, who ran a custom combine crew that McCandless worked with in South Dakota. McCandless passed along to Westerberg one of the few possessions he had retained, a much-loved 1942 edition of Tolstoy's *War and*

Peace. McCandless noted, in an inscription on the title page, that the book was being transferred to Westerberg from Alexander in October 1990. Now while the giving away of possessions was less of an issue for McCandless than receiving gifts, this nevertheless seems to contradict my argument. After all, in this example, McCandless quite emphatically marks a symbolic transaction. Then again, perhaps this, the overly explicit marking of the transaction, is itself a clue. This is clearly not the case of a spontaneously given gift; rather, it resembles a quasi-legal exchange process. It is as if, for McCandless, the exchange of gift giving brings with it an inherent risk or vulnerability, and as such, the process needs to be formalized, the symbolic transfer logged in the protective fashion of a legal contract. Differently put: if one has a solid grounding in the symbolic, then such transactions are commonplace phenomena that remain unburdened with weighty meaning or unmanageable emotionality. If one's symbolic position is, by contrast, tenuous or somehow forestalled, then it stands to reason that one might wish to restate the symbolic transaction in a definitive manner, so as to anchor the gesture and stabilize it, thus locking it into a set of clearly defined terms.

The last of the themes I foregrounded in the above case summary – the yearning for death – is, admittedly, not apparent in the published material on McCandless. This of course, may simply be the point at which the two cases most sharply diverge.[5] And, to make the point explicit, I see no reason to assume that there was anything overtly or implicitly suicidal about McCandless's excursions. It is interesting to note, however, that Krakauer's personal investment in the McCandless story stemmed from his own experiences of mountaineering, where he – and several others whom he writes about as kindred souls to McCandless – were fully aware of the mortal risks they were taking. It is intriguing to note how many of McCandless's final communications to people that he had befriended on the road (for example, Jan Burres and Wayne Westerberg) emphasized that this would be just that, his last contact prior to his walking out "into the wild".

We cannot of course know what that phrase ("into the wild") meant for McCandless, or what broader associations this signifier might have held – consciously, or unconsciously – for him. Yet there is little doubt, in reading some of the notes McCandless left behind in his journals that being back on the road was an experience of lightness, joy, of exultation at being able to live life to the full. Indeed, his references to raw existence and unfiltered experience (see Krakauer, 1996, pp. 22–23), call to mind our earlier qualification of the Lacanian death drive not as self-annihilation, but rather as surplus vitality, as libidinal enjoyment, "a desperate affirmation of life" (Lacan, 1992, p. 263). They resonate with Žižek's description of the death drive as that "excess of life [...] which persists beyond [...] (biological) life [...] [to which] humans are [...] passionately attached" (Žižek, 2006, p. 61).

Perhaps the closest we can come to an approximation of what going 'into the wild' meant for McCandless was a third-person declaration he wrote on a piece of plywood that was found inside the abandoned bus where his body was eventually discovered. In this message, he referred to himself as a voyager who had escaped the poisoning confines of civilization and succeeded in the spiritual revolution he had set for himself becoming, triumphantly, lost in the wild (Krakaeur, 1996, 163). It is worth considering such an account, in light of the following description of how certain subjects are, once pervaded by the 'undead' animation of the death drive, driven to escape the bounds of the symbolic:

> The death drive [...] does not describe literal death, but death within the symbolic order. After having rejected the symbolic order [...] the subject persists [... T]his mode of existence gives form to destruction – death in form – so that those subjects who come back to life after rejecting the symbolic universe come back anew; they are no longer the subjects who were part of the symbolic order [...] The subject enjoys being rejected by the symbolic order, enjoys refusing the enjoyment offered within the symbolic order [... However] the subject does not completely escape the symbolic order [... but] recreates it to satisfy an undying urge to continue [... T]he death drive is obsession with continuation, not death itself [...] the death drive [...] is not the cessation of life but its continuation.
>
> (Dawkins, 2015)

This is a rich passage that contains a series of ideas that helpfully illuminate the struggle with symbolic marking that both my patient and Christopher McCandless appear to have experienced, albeit in different ways. First, we should note that the death drive here is fought not primarily against the boundaries of life but against the *delimiting boundaries of the symbolic order* (social symbolic roles, transactions, exchanges, identities, etc.). In McCandless's case, one could convincingly argue that "into the wild" signified precisely this, an attempted escape from – or opposition to – a given societal form of the symbolic order. Second, defying the symbolic gives "form to destruction" for Dawkins (2015) in the sense that such defiant subjects "come back to life", and are made anew; it enables new modes of enjoyment, and an undying urge to continue. The last qualification is crucial: the death drive – and this holds both for my patient's dangerous sailing expeditions and McCandless's Alaskan adventure – is not the cessation of life, but its insistence, beyond the bounds and limits of practicality, social norms, and everyday comforts and expectations. McCandless's quest to conclude a spiritual revolution, to attain a supreme state of freedom, to never return to the corrupting influence of civilization (see Krakauer, 1996, p. 163), give articulate expression to such an interpretation of the death drive understood in such terms.

Let me refer back once more to Žižek, who offers another crucial qualification regards the Lacanian notion of the death drive:

> [W]hat the death drive strives to annihilate is not [... the] biological cycle of generation and corruption, but rather the symbolic order, the order of the symbolic pact that regulates social exchange and sustains debts, honours, obligations. The death drive is thus to be conceived against the background

of the opposition between [... the] social life of symbolic obligations, honours, contracts, debts, and its "nightly" obverse, an immortal, indestructible passion that threatens to dissolve this network of symbolic obligations.

(Žižek, 1999, p. 190)

This poses a challenge – indeed, potentially, a corrective – to how we think the death drive and melancholia alike. As we have seen, the death drive need not be viewed as a type of suicidal impetus, as a literal yearning for physical death (although, of course, such features may be clinically present in melancholic subjects). We need, by contrast, to read annihilation here in a different key, as aimed not merely at the stuff of life, but at the level of the *symbolic trace*. Intriguingly then, the Lacanian clinician should be attentive to a type of higher-order death, to the wish (indeed, *the drive*) to destroy, or less dramatically, to *evade* the constraints of the symbolic pact, to secede from the "social life of symbolic obligations, honours, contracts, debts" (Žižek, 1999, p. 190). Of course, such phenomena in and of themselves do not ensure a diagnosis of any sort – Lacanian diagnostics being based on structural rather than symptomatic features of a case – and yet they do provide an indication of the presence of the death drive, and, indeed potentially, as I have suggested above, of melancholia.[6]

In respect of this discussion of death drive, and of the type of death-in-life that melancholia so often appears to exemplify, we might note a crucial clinical imperative. This is to take seriously the idea that the melancholic is, in a qualified sense, 'already dead', having assumed an identification that drags them beneath the line separating the everyday immediacy of inter-subjective relationships from an existence in negativity. This clinical challenge is linked to a conceptual task, one usefully framed by Leader's (2008) comparison of mourning and melancholia. Whereas mourning involves the process of establishing the denial of a positive term, that is, a recognition of loss, by contrast, melancholia "involves the affirmation of a negative term ... an ever-present void to which the melancholic cannot give up his attachment to" (2008, p. 199). (Or, to put this in Freud's (1917) words: "The complex of melancholia behaves like an open wound, drawing to itself cathectic energies" (p. 253).) We might say then that, for the melancholic subject, the predicament is not merely that of confronting death *in life*, but that of *confronting life from the position of being 'already dead'*. Allowing a melancholic patient to formulate multiple variants of the state of *being 'dead'* – be it *via* experiences of estrangement, the cutting-off of emotional ties, twilight reveries, or attempts to exit the symbolic remit of everyday sociality – might be what enables them to live. One clinical aim with suicidal melancholics might thus be simply stated: to allow them to find ways of being dead, without necessarily ending their lives.

Melancholia as a mode of (a)sociality?

Interestingly, although Krakauer's (1996) *Into the Wild* has acquired fame due to its sensitive narrativization of the McCandless case, it engages also with the broader historical phenomena of young American explorers who had sought an escape from society by venturing into the wilderness. In other words, the McCandless story can be read not merely clinically or psychoanalytically but also sociologically. Krakauer calls our attention to certain communities that have succeeded in transforming an outsider status into something approaching a rudimentary social bond. The most salient example from his book (also memorably portrayed in the film) is a place simply referred to as 'the Slabs'. The site of an abandoned naval air base, the Slabs is essentially a series of concrete strips scattered around the desert that pays seasonal home to a wide cross-section of wanderers seeking to go off-grid, to escape mainstream society and live with as few societal and financial demands as possible. Krakauer is clearly of the opinion that the Slabs echoed, at a community level, McCandless's drive to break with the big Other (the symbolic, societal domain) of middle-class expectations, roles, and social mores.

The instance of self-ostracization embodied by McCandless can thus be read as symptomatic of both a culture of hyper-connectivity and an act of rupture from the tyranny of networked existence.[7] We thus approach the intriguing question of whether such communities become sites of melancholic detachment from prevailing social norms. This question is deserving of further and more developed consideration in its own right.

For the time being, let me add one further example of such a broader sociological imperative to go off-grid: A CNN report of March 2016 described a group of people living in rural Montana who sustain themselves by scavenging meat from bison carcasses left by hunters. Dubbed 'the gleaners', the community is comprised largely of people who have "left behind their urban lifestyles to pursue a more natural existence" (Neild, 2016). 'The gleaners' are "an ad hoc community of people from different backgrounds and locations who, in some cases have acquired butchery skills, quit their jobs and moved to the wilderness" (Neild, 2016). Neild's report notes – in an interesting echo with the McCandless case – that many of 'the gleaners' have assumed adopted names, to distance themselves from the life they grew up in. There are an intriguing number of parallels at the communal level with what we have seen as characteristic of melancholic subjectivity. This, the paradoxical idea of melancholia as an ostensibly asocial means of constituting a rudimentary communal bond, points to an interesting area of prospective future sociological and/or psychosocial research.

A lost object, after all?

Let me add a closing consideration. It is perhaps not insignificant that both McCandless and my patient maintained a passionate animosity toward their parents and their fathers in particular. It will not have escaped some readers that such a vitriolic relation of hate – a basis, surely, for an internalized relation of (super-ego) aggression – is evident in both the cases discussed above. Such a hated object would no doubt feature as a key emblem in a Freudian reading of the melancholic dynamics apparent in both such cases. Had we had more clinical material to work with, we might have considered whether the difficulties my patient and McCandless likewise experienced in intimate relationships might have stemmed from early childhood relationships with their respective parents. It may have been that such relationships – at first cherished, then lost and transformed into the basis of both hatred and identification – overshadowed all subsequent relationships, making them largely unworkable.

True as this may have been, my focus here has been to identify a different series of diagnostic markers, to suggest that we need not think of melancholia only within the parameters of the lost, resented, and subsequently internalized object (Freud's account), but also according to a different set of analytical priorities. These analytical and diagnostic priorities concern: difficulties in processing symbolic exchanges (receiving gifts, being locked into symbolic obligations or roles), problems in mediating intimacy (the terror of closeness, inability to place oneself relative to the desire of the Other), a yearning for anonymity and disappearance, and existence within a twilight world beyond the constraints of a given symbolic domain (a place beyond the living, a going 'into the wild'). Each of these themes, as I hope is by now clear, represents a mode of the death drive.

Notes

1   The point can be stressed by citing Lacan's declaration that "[A]s a subject, it is through his disappearance that he makes his mark" (2006f, 657).
2   It perhaps helps to add here that this distinction between the Other and that real object (object *a*) that is seemingly in them is already apparent in Freud's (1917) famous declaration that the melancholic "knows whom he has lost but not what he has lost in him" (p. 245). In fact, this distinction of Freud's was one of the origins of Lacan's notion of the object *a*.
3   A publisher's description of *The Autobiography of a Supertramp* reads as follows: "At the end of the 19th Century, W.H. Davies hustled his way across America, working when he could, begging and stealing when he couldn't. He saw life on the breadline. He was beaten up in New Orleans, thrown into prison in Michigan and was present at lynchings in Tennessee, truly a diarist of the nether side of the American dream" (see: https://www.amazon.com/The-Autobiography-of-a-Supertramp/dp/B0054LQS8S).
4   That McCandless chose to write about himself in the third person is telling. Might it be that he – like my patient – was made uncomfortable when his presence was too directly marked or affirmed? Perhaps the third-person 'he' afforded a greater modicum of distance than the intimacy implied by the first-person 'I'? Interestingly, it is precisely for this reason that literary theorist Derek Attridge (2005) argues that author J.M. Coetzee uses the third person in his autobiographical novels *Boyhood* and *Youth*.
5   There is an important and perhaps definitive difference between the two cases. My patient wished to retrospectively erase all symbolic traces of his life. McCandless, by contrast, left a note, signed, significantly, in his own full name, thanking God, offering God's blessings to all, and affirming that he had had a happy life.
6   The above discussion of the death drive does point to a useful differential diagnostic qualification. Whereas an obsessional neurotic may act out a given (repressed) conflict, repeatedly sending (an unconscious) message to the Other, a psychotic melancholic

is more likely – applying here Lacan's notion of the 'passage to the act' (2014) – to suspend any such performance for the Other preferring simply to act, breaking with the Other altogether. Building on this: whereas the obsessional would likely indulge in indecision, procrastinating and vacillation (or fantasy), the psychotically structured subject is often far more decisive, willing to take the radical step that the obsessional shirks away from. This gives a different inflection to the diagnostic indicator so often stressed in Lacanian theory: the uncertainty and ambivalence of the obsessional neurotic is to be opposed to the certainty of the psychotic. This suggests, in turn – perhaps quite obviously - that the death drive presents very differently in cases of neurosis.

7 I owe this point to Julie Walsh.

References

Attridge, D. (2005). *J.M. Coetzee and the Ethics of Reading*. Chicago: Chicago University Press.

Davies, W.H. (1908). *The Diary of a Super-tramp*. London: A.C. Fifield.

Dawkins, S. (2015). Death Drive. http://www.actforlibraries.org/death-drive/

Freud, S. (1917). Mourning and Melancholia. In J. Strachey (Ed.), *The Standard Edition of the Complete Psychological Works of Sigmund Freud, Volume XIV* (pp. 237–258). London: Hogarth Press.

Freud, S. (1923). The Ego and the Id. In J. Strachey (Ed.), *The Standard Edition of the Complete Psychological Works of Sigmund Freud, Volume XIX* (pp. 3–66). London: Hogarth Press.

Grigg, R. (2015). Melancholia and the unabandoned object. In P. Gherovici & M. Steinkoler (Eds), *Lacan on Madness: Madness, Yes You Can't* (pp. 139–158). London & New York: Routledge.

Krakauer, J. (1996). *Into the Wild*. Anchor: New York.

Lacan, J. (1992). *The Seminar of Jacques Lacan, Book VII: The Ethics of Psychoanalysis, 1959–1960*. London: W.W. Norton.

Lacan, J. (2014). *Anxiety: The Seminar of Jacques Lacan, Book X* (A. R. Price, Trans.). Cambridge: Polity Press.

Leader, D. (2003). Some Thoughts on Mourning and Melancholia. *Journal for Lacanian Studies*, *1*, 4–37.

Leader, D. (2008). *The New Black: Mourning, Melancholia and Depression*. London: Penguin.

McCandless, C. (2014). *The Wild Truth*. New York: HarperOne.

Neild, B. (2016). Montana's gleaners scavenge meat from bison carcasses left by hunters. Retrieved from http://www.cnn.com

Penn, S. (2007). (Screenplay & Director) *Into the Wild*. Los Angeles: Paramount Pictures.

Verhaeghe, P. (2001). *Beyond Gender: From Subject to Drive*. New York: Other Press.

Žižek, S. (1999). There is no sexual relationship. In Elizabeth Wright & Edmond Wright (Eds.) *The Žižek Reader* (pp. 174–205). London: Blackwell.

Žižek, S. (2006). *The Parallax View*. Cambridge, MA: MIT Press.

Chapter 8

Susan Stern

Sham

Geneviève Morel

In her memoir, Susan Stern muses: "I will grow old ungracefully, longing for the release of death and hating its insistent approach, and never really know peace" (Stern, 1975, p. 363). Few things are as troubling as the mass departure of the young people from our societies, sometimes mere teenagers, to fight a merciless war against our Western democracies, by targeting their inhabitants, the so-called *kuffars* (unbelievers), be they Muslims, Christians, Jews, or atheists. Having first emerged some years ago, this phenomenon has escalated since the declaration by the Islamic State (*Daesh*), on June 29, 2014, of a "caliphate" on the territories previously controlled by Iraq and Syria. Indoctrinated by the IS online ideologists, the "*jihadī*" fighters submit themselves to a perverted and cruel religious doctrine, which leads to mass murder and martyrdom. From one day to the next, they deny their families and their loved ones, as well as their country, which they now hate with a passion. How and why does this happen?

Despite the many sociological, psychological, and journalistic studies devoted to these questions, we are still missing a proper "clinic of terrorism" – i.e., genuine case studies. I use the somewhat controversial term "terrorism" to denote either the fact of committing violent acts against the democratic society one is living in, in order to destroy it from the inside, or because of today's "global terrorism," leaving to fight in the *jihadi* combat zones, especially in Syria or Iraq.

Some political scientists reject case studies because they rightly argue that there is no "typical profile" of a terrorist. Psychoanalysis does not believe in such "typical profiles," either – instead, it focuses on individual cases, which are always singular. However, it considers that studying a single case can, in fact, be instructive or even paradigmatic, as it gives us a glimpse of something more universal. Examining the trajectory of just one of these young people can help us shed light on some of the causes of terrorism, especially the terrorism of today.

A psychoanalyst relies on the words of those he or she listens to, and I have had the opportunity to speak, in a forensic or medical context, with a number of *jihadists* returning from Syria – those who in France have been called "*les revenants.*"[1] I then decided to read other testimonies, of terrorists from different historical periods and countries. It is worth pointing out that the practice of writing one's memoirs, which has become quite rare today, was very common throughout

DOI: 10.4324/9781003216391-9

both the 19th and 20th centuries. In France, prison directors and psychiatrists used to encourage European anarchists to write down their memories and explain their motivations, all the way to the gallows; they expected to learn something valuable for both the present and the future from these texts. For example, we have the memoirs of Émile Henry, the author of the first large-scale terrorist attack, who detonated a bomb in a busy neighborhood in Paris, as well as other anarchists. This practice survived until the second half of the 20th century and throughout the student revolts, which in many countries led to the formation of new extremist movements. A number of activists, who had gone underground for having committed acts of terrorism – especially in Germany, Italy, France and sometimes the United States – also spent their long years in prison writing their autobiographies.

As Lacan pointed out, Freud was very comfortable with autobiographic texts such as Schreber's *Memoirs*, based on which he formulated a number of crucial lessons on psychosis. Akin to the practice of free-associating in a psychoanalytic session, the author of an autobiography offers us certain thoughts, the true significance of which he sometimes ignores, and which help illuminate his life and destiny. Deciphering these writings falls under the rubric of what Freud called "applied psychoanalysis."

Of course, we cannot put the late 19th-century anarchists, 20th-century revolutionaries, and today's *jihadists* all in one bag. The context has changed and so has the style of writing. With the rise of individualism and the literary genre of *auto-fiction*, the memoirs of the young revolutionaries of the late 20th century focus much more on their personal motivations and intimate life than those of their anarchist predecessors. Some are of no use to us because they are too infiltrated by ideology, which seems to efface any grasp of subjectivity; this problem has also been observed by those who care for the imprisoned candidates for martyrdom. We could also object that autobiographies are necessarily permeated by fiction, as the contemporary label of autofiction suggests. However, this does not impede our research; in any case, as Lacan argued, truth has the structure of fiction (Lacan, 2001, pp. 12–13). The fictional parts of these memoirs can, in fact, indicate to us something about what cannot be stated directly.

Reading and deciphering these older texts can therefore tell us much about the present time; in fact, we find some of the characteristics that we might otherwise consider quite recent. For example, the phenomenon of the "born-again" converts, who leave everything overnight to blindly devote themselves to Islam, and who commit acts of terrorism in their own country or leave to fight with the IS in Syria. The anarchist Luigi Lucheni, who assassinated the Austrian Empress Sissi in Geneva at the beginning of 20th century, had "accidentally" converted to anarchism, as he himself put it, only months before his crime. Moreover, he decided to commit a regicide – *any* regicide – just a few days before killing Sissi, also nearly by accident. Before his conversion, he had been a dutiful army soldier, appreciative of the order and discipline imposed by the military – a far cry from the anarchist doctrine. As we will see, Susan Stern of the Weathermen, a revolutionary group formed in the United States in the 1960s, whose case I discuss below, also experienced such an abrupt "conversion." There are other phenomena that we can find among different extremists across space and time: youth; the importance of "fatal" couples and brotherhoods; the tendency to follow a romantic partner among women; the fierce idealism; previous dislocation; indoctrination as a reaction to the existential void; the importance of an intimate event, which then serves as a point of attraction to an ideology, and so on.

The differential importance of religion in *jihadism* should also be put in a historical perspective: the late 19th-century psychiatrist Dr. Régis, who had long conversations in prison with both Lucheni and Sante Caserio (the assassin of the French president, Sadi Carnot), believed that the religious assassinations of the past, where a king was killed in the name of the assassin's faith, stemmed from the same "morbid essence"[2] as the atheist anarchists he was listening to. In his view, their dreams, visions and discourse resembled each other in every respect (Régis, 1890).

The importance of ideals

In trying to understand what happens to some of these young people today, the memoirs of Susan Stern are highly instructive. They show us the crucial importance of the ideals (the ideal ego and the ego-ideal) and of the super-ego in youth extremism. They also make it clear that what the young woman is trying to find in the extremist ideology is a solution to a severe, and perhaps psychotic, existential divide; she is looking for an ideal image, an identity that could bring together her drives and her political ideals. She is split between her violent and sexual drives, frowned upon by her comrades, and her feminine ideal. Her example also reveals that ideology is not invincible, that the individual who submits to it must actively accept it and that it can be resisted. Lastly, her book helps us examine the urgent question of what it is that such people are looking for in extremist violence: do they wish to die in order to kill, as Robert Pape suggests (Pape, 2005),[3] or kill in order to die – i.e., is this an indirect suicide?

I was drawn to Stern's autobiography for a number of reasons, including its historical interest, because it was penned early on, soon after Stern had become involved in revolutionary politics – contrary to other Weathermen who wrote and published many years later. It, therefore, has the authenticity of a "contemporary" testimony and is free of all "political speak." As we shall see, Susan was also partially resistant to the group's ideology, even though she admired its leaders, especially women. She also insists, including it in the title of her book, on her female specificity, which, as I will show, is at the heart of her personal and neurotic problematic. This is particularly interesting, given that the Weathermen organization shared its historical moment with the birth of the feminist movements of the 1960s. It was permeated, including its name, by the 1960s pop-culture – much more so than in Europe, given that the latter originated in the United States. And Susan is, to my mind, much more emblematic of this than other actors of her time.

Weathermen (1969–1976): pop terrorism

As you may remember, the Weathermen was a revolutionary group, borrowing its name from a Bob Dylan song: "You don't need the weatherman to know which way the wind blows" ("Subterranean Homesick Blues"). The group made the song the title of its founding manifesto, written in June 1969 during a Students for a Democratic Society (SDS) convention. The ironic allusion to the imminence of revolution enabled Bernardine Dohrn, a former law student and the charismatic leader of a radical fraction of the SDS, the Revolutionary Youth Movement (RYM), to attract a bunch of SDS activists, the Weathermen. Nourished by the student revolt against the Vietnam War and racism, the SDS, sometimes called the New Left, was, at the time, 100,000 members strong.

Today, its history has been somewhat forgotten. In the beginning, SDS was founded in 1960 as the student section of the League for Industrial Democracy (LID), a liberal organization with anti-communist leanings typical of the Cold War. The SDS founders summarized their political positions in the *Port Huron Statement*, written in 1962 by Tom Hayden, the future California state senator. The statement supported the Civil Rights Movement for racial equality and condemned nuclear proliferation, but not the communists, which led to its split from the LID, which remained anti-communist. The communists, who created a group inside the SDS called the Progressive Labor Party (PLP), took part in the April 1965 March Against the Vietnam War on Washington, which brought together 15,000–20,000 students. After the march, the number of SDS members skyrocketed, reaching 100,000 in 1969. Following the Marxist-Maoist doctrine, the PLP saw the organization of the working class as its most important task; the aim of the Weathermen's June 1969 manifesto was to isolate the PLP, which was trying to take control of the SDS.

One of the burning issues faced by the SDS was the question of racism. The Black Panther movement, founded in 1966 to fight for civil rights, only included black activists. It advocated the seizure of power by the oppressed peoples around the world. Under the impetus of Malcolm X, it demanded that whites fight against their own racism; this created a split in the SDS and contributed to the hardening of its discourse. Some of its members began to read Régis Debray (*Revolution in the Revolution*) and think about the potential application, in the United States, of his foco theory, which argued that small paramilitary groups could overthrow the capitalist system from the inside. Frantz Fanon (*The Wretched of the Earth*, 1961) and Wilhelm Reich (*Mass Psychology of Fascism*, 1930–1933) were also among their key influences. The SDS journal *New Left Notes* (*NLN*) advocated overthrowing the state and abolishing private property. The 1968 assassination of Martin Luther King triggered a wave of riots throughout the country. A number of universities, including Columbia, were occupied, posing a serious challenge to the pacifism of many students.

This was also the beginning of the women's liberation movement, supported by *NLN* articles such as *Sex and Caste* by Casey Hayden and Mary King (1966) and *The Look Is You* by Bernardine Dohrn and Naomi Jaffe (1968). The year 1967 saw the formation of the first women-only groups, such as WITCH or the Redstockings.

The PL remained opposed to all deviations from classical Marxism, especially the antiracist and feminist struggles, which it saw as secondary to the class struggle. It therefore considered the Black Panther Party as reactionary, while the Weathermen wanted to learn from it. Contrary to the PLP, the authors of the Weathermen manifesto called for armed struggle, echoing the global anticolonial fight. The liberation of the African-American community, considered as an internal colony of the United States, was part of this. Hence the idea of an alliance with the Black Panthers and the North Vietnam fighters. This armed struggle was to be supported not only by working-class youth, but more largely by the white American youth affected by the "contradictions of decaying imperialism." The group's name was a wink addressed to the counter-culture of this youth, which was just beginning to invent new ways of living (communes, drug taking, group sex, non-monogamy, and so on).

On June 20, 1969, in Chicago, about a hundred SDS activists joined Bernardine Dohrn in founding the Weathermen. During this student "coup," she declared: "We are the SDS," thus endorsing the scission and the rapid dispersion of the members of the SDS, which never again recovered. The leaders of the new avantgarde included Bill Ayers from Chicago, Marc Rudd from New Jersey and Jeff Jones from California, all students from middle-class or wealthy backgrounds.

On March 6, 1970, on 11th Street in Greenwich Village, New York, there was an explosion at the Townhouse, a building owned by James Wilkerson, a rich publicist whose daughter Cathy had borrowed the house to use it as a bombmaking lab with her comrades. However, one of the bombs exploded too soon, killing the young pyro-technicians working in the basement: Cathy's lover Terry Robbins and two of his friends, Teddy Gold and Diana Oughton. Cathy Wilkerson and another activist, Kathy Boudin, who were upstairs in the house, survived the blast and managed to escape the FBI.

This is to show just how much things had accelerated in less than nine months, between the SDS split of June 1969 and the March 1970 explosion. In November 1969, the Weathermen called for three days of anti-war protest in Chicago, under the slogan "Bring the War Home!" This demonstration, the so-called "Days of Rage," became incredibly violent, with many attacks on the police and a great number of arrests. However, few students had responded to the Weathermen's appeal, showing the true collapse of the SDS.

The Black Panthers were constantly hunted by the FBI. A young activist, Fred Hampton, was killed in his bed. In late December 1969 in Flint, Michigan, the Weathermen responded by declaring a "war" against the state, thus managing to scare away other, more frightened, students. The decision to go underground in order to take up armed struggle was made official via the apocalyptic speech delivered by Dohrn, in which she went as far as to defend the murder of Sharon Tate by the Manson cult, adopting the "fork salute" of four fingers held up in the air as the Weathermen rallying sign (she later claimed her speech was meant to be ironic, but it seems that nobody at the time understood this). Before the explosion at the Townhouse in March 1970, bombs had already been planted in several cities, but miraculously no one had been killed. Policemen were an explicit target ("Off the pigs!"), together with the military, who were seen as complicit in the Vietnam War.

Although the Townhouse explosion plunged the group into a state of profound mourning, it also impelled them further toward clandestinity, as they were now pursued by the FBI. Weathermen thus became the Weather Underground Organization (WUO). Its new targets were symbolic and the police were alerted each time to avoid victims. Bernardine Dohrn announced the new strategy of "armed propaganda" (Burroughs, 2015a, p. 122)[4] via a tape recorded at a secret location. To show that the group was serious about its "Declaration of A State of War," a New York police station was bombed less than two weeks later (Berger, 2010, pp. 212–214). During the 1971–1972 period, the FBI counted more than 1,800 domestic bombings: not all of these were WUO's responsibility, because there were many other terrorist groups at the time (Burroughs, 2015b).

The majority of WUO's underground leaders gave themselves up to the FBI after 1976: the Vietnam War had ended, they had aged and had children, and, above all, they knew that the majority of the charges against them would be dropped due to procedural errors. In fact, the charges collected by the FBI's COINTELPRO program, launched by J. Edgar Hoover against domestic political movements, were pronounced illegal in 1976. Indeed, few of the Weathermen members spent time in prison, except for those who pursued their struggle with other terrorist groups and faced charges of killing policemen during the Brink's armed robbery in 1981; this was the case of Kathy Boudin, who had escaped the Townhouse explosion, and her husband David Gilbert.

Some of the WUO leaders such as Bernardine Dohrn's husband Bill Ayers became the icons of the New American Left and published their memoirs years later. However, at times, these texts seem somewhat sugar-coated.

Epiphanies and chasms

Susan Stern published her personal journal of a Weatherwoman in 1976, a year before she died from an overdose at the age of 33. Her memoir is rarely mentioned among the books of the New Left and the Weathermen.[5] It tells the story of a tragic drifting, a fragile person who was drawn, in the name of a political ideology, into a violent movement that eventually destroyed her. Incarcerated after the violent events of 1970–1971, Stern spent her days in prison writing a detailed account of the previous years, first as a member of the SDS and later the Weathermen, spanning the period of 1966–1972 and published a year before her death.

She speaks about herself candidly; her story is written in chronological order like a logbook, fresh like a snapshot. As a regular member of the movement, she is not trying to justify the political strategy over which she had no say. Because she never reached the highest echelons of the group's hierarchy, she offers us, without any clichés, a glimpse of its life quite different from that of its leaders – Cathy Wilkerson, Bill Ayers, Marc Rudd or others – who wrote their memoirs sometimes decades after the events (Ayers, 2001; Rudd, 2009; Wilerson, 2007).

Together with her then-husband, Robby Stern, Susan became a member of the SDS in August 1967; she was 24 years old. The couple's relationship had been floundering and they were looking for a fresh start. After having both studied at Syracuse and Susan teaching in a ghetto school, they left the East Coast in 1966 and moved to Seattle; Robby enrolled in a law school and Susan began a degree in social work. Although she did not have much faith in the project, she was hoping to save their marriage and escape a "drab, miserable existence." She felt inferior to her gifted husband and resented the fact that, in student meetings, she was generally known simply as "Robby Stern's wife."

It is Robby who offers her the first joint: in a kind of exaggerated premonition, she thinks that smoking marijuana will lead to insanity and death. On the same day, she kicks Robby out, but keeps the weed. Separated from Robby and feeling very depressed, she meets a group of hippies at a demonstration. She writes: "For the first time in my life, I felt I belonged somewhere" (Stern, 1975, pp. 11, 14). This verdict marks a fleeting joy of having found a place. However, she quickly falls back into her depression. In fact, the entire diary oscillates between moments of losing and finding herself; each time, she has the sense of having been reborn as a new person, yet these moments grow increasingly rarer.

Her encounter with the budding women's liberation movement inspires such enthusiasm in her that she starts a feminist group in Seattle as part of the SDS. In the group, she learns to speak to and be listened to by other women. She adopts a new style: she changes her glasses, wears bright red lipstick and a miniskirt. "I developed my Style. Zip, zap, I was a new Susan Stern" (Stern, 1975, pp. 21–22). The alternation accelerates: each brief moment of euphoria leads to a deep feeling of loss, followed by the emergence of destructive fantasies and visions. Below are two typical examples.

One: after successfully graduating from her Master's program in Seattle, Susan finds a well-paid job as a go-go dancer in San Francisco. She is happy, but immediately becomes obsessed with a morbid fantasy. She imagines reading the newspaper headlines: a girl like her (from New Jersey) is found dead, strangled in her topless dancer costume.

Two: at the large SDS demonstration in August 1968, during the Democratic Convention in Chicago, Susan feels "part of a great whole" (Stern, 1975, pp. 20, 34, 36). Feeling vindictive, she is "ready to riot": "I wanted to kill." When she is injured during the demonstration, she has terrible, quasi-hallucinatory visions, like epiphanies: she sees the dead body of Malcolm X, the lynchings of black Americans, and Vietnamese babies covered with napalm.

I thought about Auschwitz, and mountains of corpses piled high in the deep pits dug by German Nazis. I closed my eyes tightly, but tears oozed from under my lids and rolled off my face. A new feeling was struggling to be born in me. It had no name, but it made me want to reach beyond myself to others who were suffering. I felt real, as if suddenly I had found out something true about myself [...] . Now I would fight.

On both occasions, she describes her body as a "corpse." In the second vision, she enters a state of universal communion with all the victims of genocides and Nazism. However, it is paradoxically precisely this identification, this communion with the dead, that brings her out of her depression, provoking feelings of elation and sustaining her desire to keep fighting.

My super-ego nickname

When the SDS splits in June 1969, Susan follows the Weathermen. She feels galvanized by the charismatic Bernardine Dohrn, although she misses the "big family" of the SDS and the feeling of belonging it gave her. She asks herself whether the split is a "suicide," but concludes that:

listening to Bernardine, I felt that I had finally connected with my own personal destiny; that I had a place, a function in life. That place was with the Weathermen, that function was to fight for the revolution to the best of my ability [...] Weatherman. I fell in love with a concept. [...] I ceased to think of Susan Stern as a woman; I saw myself as a revolutionary tool. [...] my family, my past all faded into dreary insignificance. For the first time in my life that I could remember, I was happy.

(Stern, 1975, p. 72)

In her descriptions, we always find the same conjunction of a happy *rebirth* – which is reaffirmed each time, as if it was the first time – and a correlative *loss* of the ego and its possessions, where even her feminine identity becomes untenable.

In late 1969, during a demonstration into which she throws herself with abandon, Susan suffers a severe concussion and needs to be hospitalized. Her singular style is not appreciated by Weathermen leaders, despite her efforts at self-criticism to obey their iron discipline. She then gives herself a derisory nickname – Susan Stern *Sham* (Stern, 1975, pp. 191, 208). In her self-baptism, the self-derisory sobriquet materializes her super-ego's agreement with the leaders' critique.

The Freudian super-ego is a paradoxical concept: its power is fueled by the guilt generated not just by actions, but also by unconscious wishes (Freud, 1930, pp. 57–146). In addition, the misfortunes suffered by the ego and its renunciations are considered as faults and provoke further punishment by the super-ego, which can then lead to actions against the law. The super-ego gradually becomes more and more ferocious; it expands, fueled by the death drive and destructiveness unbound from the erotic libido. When Susan is disparaged and punished during the criticism sessions, not only does she accept her punishment, but her super-ego amplifies it further – hence the adoption of this intimate nickname, a sign of her downfall. Still, she remains with the Weathermen, even though she has been quarantined. The leaders eventually exclude her completely when they decide, in December 1969 in Flint, to go underground. Susan hopes to re-enter the organization, but instead falls into a deep depression.

In spite of this, the hope for a new rebirth never leaves her. In March 1970, she reads about the Townhouse explosion, just after her divorce from Robby has been finalized. She decides to go underground with another small revolutionary group, the Seattle Liberation Front, but eventually changes her mind. In a moment of despair, wishing to end with it all, she collects her old letters and notebooks, her poems and photos from her youth, and, together with the beautiful clothes her father had given her, throws everything away:

> Soon there would be no more Susan Stern. She would be dead, and the person she had been would have another face, another color hair, another name, another past. She would invent it, build it, engineer it to be exactly what she wanted it to be, what she had never been. […] A past of fiction, a life of science fiction. Susan Stern Sham would end finally, finally she would end.
>
> (Stern, 1975, p. 249)

To sacrifice everything: her possessions, her ego, her image, her female identity and, finally, even her name and nickname. And, *in fine*, her life. The perpetual repetition of these losses seems to be the necessary precondition for the glimmering and vain hope of a mythical reconstruction, not just of the present, but also of her past.

Dream-o-lution[6]

But it is not yet 1970. Previously, Susan is passionately devoted to her revolutionary beliefs, but also remains lucid, as if she was not completely taken in by the Weathermen propaganda – a contradiction that contrasts with the blind obedience of her fellow activists.

Constantly concerned about her femininity, she is particularly interested in the new feminist movements such as the National Organization of Women (NOW). She has a hard time tolerating the dominance of certain male leaders, who abuse the so-called *sleeping rule* (everyone must sleep with everyone) to bend their female comrades to their will. Although she feels attracted to the "great" leader Bill Ayers, she refuses to go to bed with him, because he behaves too much like a "superstar" (Stern, 1975, p. 76). Still, she feels obliged to sleep with a certain "JJ," simply because he saved her from the cops. She becomes more resistant to the "Crush Monogamy" slogan when she finds a regular lover, Garrity, with whom she also does drugs. Unfortunately, Garrity is not part of the Weathermen.

Some leaders are dismissive of her – for example, Marc Rudd. The loudmouths always win: "There was no way to escape the fact that I was white, female, from a wealthy family, Jewish, had been married, was well educated, had been a ghetto school-teacher, etc. The obvious reaction to Rudd's contempt for me never crossed my mind; he was from a similar background" (Stern, 1975, pp. 42-43). She also struggles with the criticism of another leader, Kathy Boudin, who sidelines her, even though Susan does her best to perform various menial tasks in order to be accepted: "She frightened me to death. [...] Kathy seemed above sexual need, beyond the petty and childish fantasies I still secreted about falling in love and being loved" (Stern, 1975, p. 59). At the same time, she is not blind to the barely disguised *jouissance* that these admirers of Mao's Red Guards derive from the criticism sessions they impose on others.

Susan dreams of the big day to come: "In my dreams of revolution was a world where class and race had vanished, and only peace, love and happiness remained" (Stern, 1975, pp. 62, 66, 68, 69). Yet her dream is crushed by the collapse of the SDS. There were 500,000 of them in the United States, a big community open to everyone, but all that ended with the "Big Split. Not immediately. But inevitably. [...] Pig paranoia became a plague." Even though she has followed Bernardine Dohrn with great enthusiasm, Susan looks toward the future without any illusions. Also, she has no say over it. "I wandered away from the Seattle group with a growing sense of alarm and isolation. Somehow the die had been cast, the split was on, but did I personally want it? It had nothing to do with me, really. I was just a plebeian; the leadership had made the decision, and now it was a fact. How was I related to this fact?"

At the same time, she is not ready to obey blindly. After one last criticism session, when she is reproached for her eccentricity, her drug habits and above all the shocking contradiction between her revolutionary feminist ideals and having earned her living as a go-go dancer, the Weathermen Seattle collective decides to exclude her from the local leadership. When she is invited to come back shortly afterward, she refuses. She wants to stay in the group but keep her freedom: "I was a Weatherman cheerleader. I was a religious zealot. I was a crazy fool in love with the notion of revolution without any idea of its concept" (Stern, 1975, pp. 96, 123). She believes that the Weathermen destroy instead of constructing; she does not want to submit. She concludes: "As much as I loved Weatherman, I loved my individuality more." She keeps her high heels and her miniskirt; she still refuses to adhere to the sleeping rule. She accepts her contradictions. She even consents to the criticism sessions enforced by the leadership, because she believes that transformation can be achieved at the cost of losing oneself. However, does she not already indulge in this type of process on her own? Despite her fascination with the leaders she admires, she knows very well they are mistaken and refuses to join in what she considers abuse. Perhaps Susan Stern is a sham, but she is not just a pawn.

Suicides on repeat

Susan's ex-husband Robby decided to never follow the Weathermen. He would mock them, asking her ironically if they were planning to kill all white

Americans. He admonishes her right from the start: "You didn't start seeing things that way when you became a revolutionary. You have always done these numbers behind suicide." In his view, the Weathermen simply provided a social and political pretext to Susan's pre-existing suicidal tendencies (Stern, 1975, p. 98).

Indeed, Susan speaks about a series of suicide attempts during her childhood. When she was 3 years old, her mother, "beautiful and childlike," left the family home for another man, whom she loved "more than her children." Susan and her younger brother Roger were thus separated from their mother at a very young age. After a brutal legal battle that lasted six years, the custody of the children was given to the father, a rich businessman who adored and spoiled his daughter. It is evident that Susan perceived the mother's leaving as an abandonment and that this was constantly emphasized to her by her father.

In this dramatic context, Susan first attempted suicide at the age of 13. Her father slaps her because he thinks that he saw her in a car with her mother. This is not true and the girl, who is suffering greatly from the separation, answers that she has not seen her mother for months. The father does not believe her; in response, she swallows an overdose of pills (Stern, 1975, pp. 230–231). Susan speaks about this first attempt when she describes another, in late 1969, after the Weathermen convention and the "declaration of a state of war" in Flint, a time when she felt "untouchable." During one of the endless criticism sessions, she is asked, in order to free herself from her bourgeois upbringing, to sleep with a couple she likes. She cannot comply. In addition, the sudden decision of the Weathermen to go underground in order to take up arms leaves her speechless: she refuses to leave the world in this way. Overnight, she is then kicked out of her small local Weathermen community. "And then I got the idea. Suicide! […] . And here I was at the age of 27, still as emotionally unequipped to deal with myself as I was at 13." Feeling transformed into a "worm, disgusting, foul," she swallows a lethal dose of Seconal, a dangerous barbiturate. By pure chance, her lover, Garrity, finds her unconscious and saves her. It is no coincidence that her autobiography makes a connection between these two suicide attempts: the first has to do with being let down by the mother, which is confirmed by the father. The second is a repetition of this abandonment by the Weathermen leadership, which, for her, functions as the law.

This is the beginning of Susan's desperate and suicidal drifting from one group to another. Looking for an alternative to the Weathermen, she joins another group, Sundance, named after the film *Butch Cassidy and the Sundance Kid*, the very same that inspired the desire to "go out in a blaze of glory" in Teddy Robbins, the bomb-maker of Townhouse. The members of Sundance practice a kind of "festival of *jouissance*." Occasionally, Susan also spends time with another revolutionary group, the SLF, where she sleeps with any man available and takes a lot of drugs.

She falls into a spiral of violence. With her comrades, she prepares "The Day After" in Chicago, a demonstration to protest the trial against a group of demonstrators, the "Chicago Seven," seen as unjust. Susan hopes that she will get herself killed:

> I was obsessed with death and dying. I began to think about bombing the police station again, making sure I perished in the explosion. I fantasized about shootouts with a dozen pigs, killing some of them, and finally getting killed myself. I daydreamed of setting an ROTC building on fire, and burning to death in the blaze. My death had to count for something. I couldn't just die anymore; I had to die with meaning. My life couldn't be wasted by a wasted death. In those days before TDA, I was consumed with murder and suicide and violence.
>
> (Stern, 1975, pp. 236, 237, 241, 244)

However, after this post-demonstration, the Sundance leaders exclude her from their group as well, describing her behavior as "kamikaze." Susan is still excited by the sound of the broken windows. When she hears about the Townhouse explosion, she experiences a wave of self-hatred at the idea of still being alive: "I hated my flesh, my breath, my nose, my feet. I despised the tenacity with which I clung to it. My thoughts swung even more morbidly. If one could not live meaningfully, one at least could die meaningfully. That much control one had over one's life." In other words, she downright envies the three Townhouse victims.

As her husband said, Susan Stern had had suicidal aspirations since childhood; these then morphed into her revolutionary ideas and quickly became accentuated. As we have seen, she even dreams about being killed with a gun in her hand. During the Days of Rage, she carries a revolver and learns how to make Molotov cocktails. After her trial in 1970, she leaves for the mountains with a chemist, to learn how to handle dynamite. She speaks about her visions of blowing up the IBM and Boeing factories: "We hated America. [...] . Our hearts were in the hills, with our bombs; our hearts were underground, with the Weathermen" (Stern, 1975, p. 271). Susan would like to give her own death the same revolutionary meaning as the one she ascribes to the Townhouse victims. At the same time, this idea and practice of violence animate and galvanize her, keeping her alive like a regular dose of speed: the planned death is thus suspended each time, but for how long?

The Weatherwoman: how to heal the fatal flaw?

Stern is able to formulate the division that is gnawing at her: "My sexual desires came from a different part of me than my revolutionary ideals." Faced with this split between her sexual drives and her ideals, she feels terribly alone (Stern, 1975, p. 252). During the summer of 1970, she tries to put this division into action, on one hand, through rampant bodily practice: "sex, dope and violence!" is her slogan; on the other hand, by devoting the rest of her time to the secret implementation of her revolutionary project – i.e., making reliable bombs. However, this solution is not quite satisfying.

Susan tries to overcome the division she could not assume in different ways. First, she tries to conceal it by the "ideal image" of the female revolutionary, Bernardine Dohrn, whom she has admired since their first meeting in the SDS: "The way she spoke and moved; such control, such self-assurance, such elegance. She immediately became a symbol of what I hoped to become. At the same time, I felt helplessly inadequate in the face of all that splendor" (Stern, 1975, p. 47).

The desire to serve a political cause cannot be separated from a certain conformism vis-à-vis the avant-garde, an attitude that can be traced back to childhood. Already as infants, we can sense our parents' expectations. These eventually form an "ego-ideal," a reference point that we use to transform our ego into an "ideal ego," the image that will satisfy the parents. The coupling between the ego-ideal and the ideal ego (Freud, 1914, pp. 67–102) functions throughout life: in the family, at school, in the army, at university, at work, in the couple, and so on. Each time, the subject tries to identify with the ideal ego defined by the elder or the boss, by the loved, envied or admired person who embodies the ego-ideal. And, each time, the success of this identification coincides with the feelings of exaltation experienced as being freed from the "ordinary yokes" of the past.

Bernardine is therefore the ideal ego before whom Susan inevitably feels miserable. During the Days of Rage they are arrested together. Even after being thrown into the police van, Bernardine retains her charm:

> She looked like a fashion model. Short black leather jacket, nice slacks, neat purple blouse, the boots – everything just so. […] I just plainly stared at her, unable to fathom the source of her charisma. She possessed a splendor all of her own. Like a queen, her nobility set her apart from other women.
>
> (Stern, 1975, pp. 150, 151, 268)

Later, Susan listens, transfixed, to the diva's first underground communique: "It was like a voice from heaven, from the future, a voice that no American law could silence." She is also impressed by other women, such as the beautiful Cathy Wilkerson, who takes the time to listen to her life story – as opposed to her mother, to whom Susan could never explain anything, given how much the mother was preoccupied with her own problems. Or, in a negative way, Kathy Boudin, who galvanizes her during a demonstration, but later turns very critical toward her and whose militant rigidity "frightens [Susan] to death" (Stern, 1975, p. 59). The feminine ideal thus becomes the sarcastic voice of the super-ego.

The other way of stitching together the two sides of her division would be, of course, to try to embody the ideal image of the leader herself. Yet Susan cannot succeed at this; her division deepens and inexorably tears her apart. When she tries to be a "serious revolutionary," she imagines herself covered in blood on the streets of Chicago. During the Days of Rage, which are broadcast on TV in "gory Technicolor," she thinks: "The whole world is watching [me]" (Stern, pp.

136–137). However, this image of a fighter again gives way to the sexy image of the go-go dancer, who is rejected by other Weatherwomen, because she stands for the objectified woman, at odds with their revolutionary ideals. As we already know, this eventually leads to Susan's exclusion, because her behavior is excessive on both fronts – on the side of the struggle and the side of femininity.

Nevertheless, she does have one opportunity to mend this inner breach, by bringing her image as a woman and a Weathermen fighter together: during the Seattle Seven hearing, a trial against a group of anti-war activists, where she is one of the defendants. She feels very important, having become *the* female voice of the revolution. She is the "lone woman defendant" and identified as such "a hundred times" by the press: "Suddenly I was someone. [...] . And finally, no one but me to undertake the tremendous responsibility of being the female voice which would be carried to other women across the country" (Stern, 1975, pp. 260, 264). Since all the top Weatherwomen have gone underground after the Townhouse explosion, "it was my voice which would be heard at rallies, mine in classrooms, mine in newspaper interviews, radio talk shows, and over the news. [...] since I had been singled out by the government, other women wanted to know what knew." Susan has found a mission. During this period, she becomes friends with Annie Anderson, a devoted activist who supports her during the ensuing difficult months, in the course of which she suffers from various physical issues: STDs, an unwished-for (and long denied) pregnancy, an incurable cold, the effects of her drug use, etc.

Thanks to this new (imposed) mission, Susan manages to take on the ideal image of the revolutionary woman. She is preoccupied with what to wear to the hearings; she alternates: "between my long black skirt and black hat and knitting like Madame De Farge [the *tricoteuse* of the French Revolution in Dickens's *A Tale of Two Cities*], and my miniskirt for a little shock therapy." In this outfit, she manages to plead and also deliver a political speech, despite the judge's attempts at preventing her from doing so.

However, the relief brought by the unifying image of the female revolutionary is short-lived. Susan quickly falls back into depression and drugs – evidence that she is not a paranoiac, because no mission seems to sustain her for very long.

She then decides – this is her third attempt at healing her split – to write her memoirs, starting in the prison where she has been sentenced for six months. She describes her mental state to her friend Anne:

> Still, I am unhappy in my role as a revolutionary, because it is not enough for me; I want to stand out in the history I am trying to make. My existence will have meaning only if lots of others know about it. Call it fame, immortality, call it what you will, until I have it, I will always be unhappy. I guess that's the saddest thing about me, my *fatal flaw*.
>
> (Stern, 1975, p. 363, emphasis added)

However, writing is not enough to stabilize her, although she manages to publish her memoirs in 1975. A year later, after another romantic disappointment, she dies from an overdose in what seems to be a barely concealed suicide. Her political adventure was born from the breakdown of her marriage to Robby; she kills herself after her latest romantic failure. The story comes full circle, especially if we think of her abandonment, as a young child, by her mother, her suicidal attempt at 13, linked to the pain of this separation, and what she was looking for later among women – namely, an ideal, but also someone who listens, which her own mother was never able to do (we have seen that she mentions this when speaking about Cathy Wilkerson). She also writes to Anne: "Love, I almost hate the word. I have always been an abysmal failure at it. I have always thought if I could find love I would not crave fame so, but it seems I lose on both scores."

Today like yesterday?

Susan Stern's activist and terrorist trajectory seems paradigmatic of the youthful appetence for the excitement of extremism and the swift passage to the act. In her case, we can indeed speak of terrorism, despite her modest discretion regarding her acts, probably due to the risks of legal persecution: when her book was published in 1975, the Weathermen were still active underground and carrying out bomb attacks. Although she does not say very much about this, Susan nevertheless mentions that she continues to make explosives and that she carries guns during demonstrations – presumably to use them.

Her political engagement was serious, even though she always trailed behind those she depended on (her husband and later Bernardine Dohrn) and never devoted herself to studying revolutionary texts (she says that she barely skimmed through the Weathermen manifesto). However, she never agreed to submit herself to the rules that bothered her, such as "Smash Monogamy," nor did she conform to stereotyped gender behavior. This ambivalence shows us that action can be prompted by an image rather than a theorized political engagement and, even though one does not quite agree, with one's leaders. Today's terrorists are often described as radical individuals completely at one with their ideology; yet, in reality, they can be ambivalent; they might hesitate for a long time, before suddenly carrying out their mad acts. Susan is a good illustration of this type of behavior.

Finally, it is the ideal image of the female revolutionary that magnetizes her, that is her "divine inspiration" – the woman she meets and whom she would like to become (Stern, 1975, p. 112). For a brief moment this image heals the painful split between her drives and her ideals, by condensing the violence that inhabits her with her ideal. The image of the revolutionary woman makes her a "passionate idealist," a term coined in 1913 by the French psychiatrist Maurice Dide (2006).

Her revolutionary involvement seems to resemble that of other students of her generation: protesting the Vietnam War and racism. However, it is based on a singular constellation.

During one demonstration, as she is getting ready to fight against the "Nazi state," ready to kill and be killed, Susan has a fleeting thought of her father. The source of her torment is her suspicion that this rich, Jewish capitalist had learned nothing "from the massacre of six million Jewish human beings in Germany" (Stern, 1975, p. 135). Susan thinks of her father as a racist who hates people of color and other religions. We remember her vision of a pile of bodies, in the sinister communion with all of the victims of genocides and of Nazism, which led her to experience herself as a corpse. From now on, Susan is situated alongside these massacred victims, while her father, who, in a sense, has foreclosed his Jewish origins, is located on the other Side – of the white men she is fighting against, the killers, the pigs. Susan also blames her father's cruelty for her suicide attempt at 13. However, at the same time, she remains her father's daughter, claiming her white bourgeois and Jewish origins. She brings all of these identities together and does not deny either of them: on one hand, she identifies as a victim of a massacre; on the other, she is the killer of white men, of pigs like her father. This further strengthens her sense of guilt.

Because of the latter, she obeys the punitive super-ego that pushes her to go kamikaze in *a version that is above all suicidal*: rather than killing, she wants to be killed, but only as long as she finds a glorious death. Her super-ego, precociously engendered by the void of her mother's abandonment, which the father did not manage to make up for, is feminine and lawless. It takes on the seductive traits of the great Weatherwomen, in fact capricious superwomen like Bernardine Dohrn or Kathy Boudin. Susan's constant preoccupation with her image and reputation resembles the concerns of other terrorists such as Terry Robbins, whose glorious end – "dying in a blaze of glory," as in the final scene of *Butch Cassidy and the Sundance Kid* – she envies.

Notes

1 After the bestselling book by the French journalist David Thomson.
2 Of course we do not believe in the existence of any such "morbid essence" – it is a term of 19th-century psychiatry.
3 According to Pape, even in 2001 the kamikaze fighters continue to commit altruistic suicides in Durkheim's sense – they sacrifice themselves for the benefit of others and a political cause.
4 For the Weatherman's Declaration of A State of War see: www.youtube.com/watch?v=jbpTvkpZluk
5 She is not at all mentioned in, for example, the books by Dan Berger, Cathy Wilkerson or Bill Ayers, even though the latter two were her comrades.
6 *Rêve-lution* in the original.

References

Ayers, B. (2001). *Fugitive Days: A Memoir*. New York: Penguin Books.
Berger, D. (2010). *Weather Underground. Une histoire explosive du plus célèbre groupe radical américain*. Paris: L'échappée.
Burroughs, B. (2015a). *Days of Rage, American's Radical Underground, the FBI and the Forgotten Age of Revolutionary Violence*. New York: Penguin Books.
Burroughs, B. (2015b, March 29). Meet the weather underground's bomb guru. *Vanity Fair*.

Dide, M. (1913/2006). *Les idealists passionnés*. Paris: Frison Roche.

Dohrn, B. and Jaffe, N. (1968). *The Look Is You: Toward a Strategy for Radical Women*. Ann Arbor: Women's Liberation.

Freud, S. (1914). 'On Narcissism', In J. Strachey (Ed.), *The Standard Edition of the Complete Psychological Works of Sigmund Freud* Volume 14. London: The Hogarth Press and the Institute of Psycho-Analysis, pp. 67–102.

Freud, S.(1930). 'Civilization and Its Discontents', In J. Strachey (Ed.), *The Standard Edition of the Complete Psychological Works of Sigmund Freud* Volume 21. London: The Hogarth Press and the Institute of Psycho-Analysis, pp. 57–146.

Lacan, J. (2001). *Litturaterre. Autres écrits*. Paris: Seuil.

Pape, R. A. (2005). *Dying to Win, The Strategic Logic of Suicide Terrorism*. New York: Random House.

Regis, E. (1890). *Les régicides dans l'histoire et dans le présent: étude medico-psychologique*. Paris: A. Maloine.

Rudd, M. (2009). *My Life with the SDS and the Weathermen Underground*. New York: William Morrow.

Stern, S. (1975). *With the Weathermen: The Personal Journal of a Revolutionary Woman*. New Brunswick: Rutgers University Press.

Wilkerson, C.P. (2007). *Flying Close to the Sun. My Life and Time as a Weatherman*. New York: Seven Stories Press.

Chapter 9

Excessive creativity in melancholia

Leon S. Brenner

The examination of the relationship between creativity and depression dates back to the days of Aristotle. In his *Problemata* (1927), Aristotle wondered why so many of the prominent figures renowned in the arts, sciences, politics, and philosophy in Ancient Greece also appeared to be depressed. The first modern scholar to examine the relationship between creativity and depression was Cesare Lombroso (1895), an Italian criminologist and physician of the 19th century who claimed that genius is one of the many forms of insanity. Nowadays, there are a vast amount of studies that attest to the existence of a relationship between creativity and depression. These include biographical studies that investigate the psychological and emotional states of famously creative individuals (Post, 1996; Jamison, 1997); psychometrical studies that examine cognitive capacities such as emotional intelligence, divergent thinking, and creative problem-solving among depressive patients (Silvia *et al.*, 2010; Salguero *et al.*, 2012); genetic studies enquiring into the co-determinacy of common genetic factors in creative and depressed people (Prentky, 2001; Chruszczewski, 2014); neuroimaging studies examining the spatial overlap in the activity in several regions of the brain during creative activity and depressed mood (Carhart-Harris *et al.*, 2008); and pharmacological studies which consider the effect of antidepressant treatment on creativity (Opbroek, 2002; Price *et al.*, 2009). All of these studies, and many more, suggest that creativity and depression are strongly correlated.

Creativity has no exclusive form of behavioral or psychiatric standardization. Nevertheless, in the past, many researchers in the field of psychology have attempted to define it exhaustively (Ludwig, 1992; Oremland, 1997; Runco & Jaeger, 2012; Kharkhurin, 2014; Weisberg, 2015; Corazza, 2016). Sigmund Freud never provided an exhaustive psychoanalytic definition of creativity. However, in the Standard Edition of the complete psychological works of Freud, one can immediately see the influence that the field of creative arts had on him, beginning with his observations on Oedipus Rex, to his allusions to Shakespeare and Goethe, to his paper on Leonardo da Vinci and Michelangelo's Moses, and many others as well. It was Freud's followers who, after his death, developed psychoanalytic theories of creativity. One might note here the work of Melanie Klein, who developed a theory of creativity in her paper "Infantile anxiety-situations

DOI: 10.4324/9781003216391-10

reflected in a work of art and in the creative impulse" (1929). Klein described creativity as an impulse to repair the object that, in the schizoid paranoid phase, had been attacked and split into good and bad. Donald Winnicott also put great emphasis on the notion of creativity in his work. In his book *Playing and Reality* (1971), he developed a theory of creativity that described it as an inherent feature of the psyche, which plays a facilitative role in psychic development and reaches far beyond the production of works of art.

This chapter will provide a Lacanian psychoanalytic interpretation of the relationship between creativity and depression. To do so, there will first be an explication of the psychoanalytic understanding of melancholia (i.e., psychotic depression) following Freud's paper "Mourning and Melancholia" (1917) and Jacques Lacan's commentaries on this text. Following this exposition, a Lacanian interpretation of creativity will be presented in terms that comply with the afore-mentioned framework. Both mourning and melancholia will then be described as creative endeavors and distinguished on the basis of the objects that condition their unique modes of creativity. Finally, new prospects for the psychoanalytic treatment of melancholia which harness its creative nature will be presented.

Melancholia in Freud and Lacan

Major depression is commonly defined as a prevalent psychiatric disorder that is characterized by persistent and pervasive depressed mood, anhedonia, a sense of worthlessness, and cognitive impairment (APA, 2013). Studies show that between 10–20% of people worldwide experience a major depressive episode in their life-time (Lim *et al.*, 2018), many of whom suffer from multiple recurring episodes and come to be at risk of suicide (Bulloch *et al.*, 2014). Many studies have iden-tified a variety of psychological, cognitive, biological, and neural mechanisms involved in the pathogenesis of major depression (Frantom & Sherman, 1999; Chávez-Eakle *et al.*, 2006; Kupfer *et al.*, 2012). However, while empirical data and the various forms of its clinical application abound, there is still no current, single, meta-psychological framework that establishes the mental causality under-lying the multiple symptoms and perspectives of major depression.

When Lacanian psychoanalysts engage with the meta-psychology of major depression, they commonly associate it with what Freud called "melancholia" and Lacan sometimes called "melancholic depression" (Lacan, 1992, p. 116). As is advanced in many chapters of this book, for Lacanian psychoanalysts, melan-cholia can be designated more precisely within the broader structure of psychosis.

In his paper, "Mourning and Melancholia" (1917), Freud developed a meta-psychological framework that establishes the psychic causality underlying melan-cholia in analogy to the fundamental characteristics of mourning. Mourning is a normative psychological process, which usually comes after the loss of someone close. This process is accompanied by an emotional state of grief, entailing a gradual emotional detachment from the lost person, and eventually freeing the mourner to find other interests and continue with their life (McGraw-Hill, 2002).

When Freud (1917) addressed the notion of mourning, he did so on the basis of his economic model of the psyche, describing it in terms of libidinal investment. Freud claimed that mourning is a process preconditioned by the loss of a major object of libidinal investment—the love object. He added that the loss of the love object is experienced by the subject as a sudden freeing-up of an excess of uninvested libidinal charge—previously invested in the love object—which is then forced to reallocate. This process unravels as a libidinal investment in the lost love object is slowly diverted to other objects thereafter taking the place of the object that was lost (p. 245). This manifests in the creation of new substitutional ties between the energy previously invested in the lost love object and other apparent objects in the vicinity of the subject's imaginary or symbolic world. When the work of mourning is complete, newly derived libidinal ties are established, and the subject can be considered to "have succeeded in freeing its libido from the lost object" (p. 252).

In the same paper, Freud went on to characterize the inner working of melancholia in direct homology to his economic model of mourning. He claimed that, like mourning, melancholia is initialized by a loss of a love object and entails the attempted recovery from this loss through the reallocation of the libidinal energy previously invested in it. However, Freud emphasized that in opposition to mourning—in which the loss of the object is consciously discernible—melancholia involves a loss of an unconscious, non-existent, or ideal object; a fact that made Freud designate it as a form of "pathological mourning" (p. 251). Freud's description of the loss of the object in melancholia is worth quoting at length:

> [In melancholia], one cannot see clearly what it is that has been lost, and it is all the more reasonable to suppose that the patient cannot consciously perceive what he has lost either. This, indeed, might be so even if the patient is aware of the loss that has given rise to his melancholia, but only in the sense he knows whom he has lost but not what he has lost in him. This would suggest that melancholia is in some way related to an object-loss which is withdrawn from consciousness, in contradistinction to mourning, in which there is nothing about the loss that is unconscious.
>
> (p. 245)

In melancholia, according to Freud, the subject experiences a unique kind of loss that, like mourning, entails an excess of uninvested libidinal charge. However, the fact that the object itself is indiscernible, from the point of view of consciousness, makes the subsequent compensatory process impossible; namely, because the lost object is undistinguishable, it is impossible to find a suitable replacement for it, and libidinal energy, freed up by its apparent loss, cannot be reallocated. Therefore, while mourning usually comes to a timely end, melancholia persists as a lasting process of unaccomplished reallocation of libidinal energy.

Freud claimed that the failure to find a suitable replacement for libidinal investment causes these excess psychic energies to be directed inwardly and become pathologically invested in the ego, thus narcissistically identifying the ego with the lost object (p. 249). Therefore, while in mourning, loss is experienced in regard to a specified lost love object, in melancholia, the lack of a lost object is translated to a loss in regard to the ego (p. 247). In this form of narcissistic regression, the ego is debased and scrutinized, resulting in what is sometimes described today as major depression (pp. 248, 251). Freud argued that, in mourning, it is the world that becomes poor and empty while, in melancholia, it is the ego itself. He added that, as a result, melancholic subjects perceive themselves as worthless, unworthy, incapable of achievement, and despicable. They experience a persistent and pervasive increase in introspection, accompanied by a sense of worthlessness and a decreased interest in the outside world (p. 244). They lose sleep, refuse to eat, and sometimes no longer wish to keep on living (p. 246). These are all psychological characteristics that today, under certain conditions, warrant a diagnosis of major depression (APA, 2013).

Lacan discusses Freud's "Mourning and Melancholia" (1917) in several of his seminars. When doing so, Lacan stresses that Freud engages with these themes in terms of relations between psychic objects (Lacan, 2019, p. 335). On the one hand, Freud generally describes the object of mourning as an important person, one's country, liberty, or ideals (Freud, 1917, p. 243). On the other hand, Freud describes the object of melancholia as being unconscious, non-existent, or ideal (p. 245).

Lacan offers a more comprehensive account of the nature of the objects of mourning and melancholia, arguing that it is only through their clear distinction that the radical difference between these two processes can be revealed (Lacan, 2014, p. 335). In order to accentuate the nature of the object of mourning, Lacan focuses on the loss of someone who was close to the subject. When doing so, he insists that this person is not necessarily a positive figure that had been loved by the subject (p. 141); for instance, it could be a person someone really hates. In formulating it in this way, Lacan preserves Freud's definition of the love object as determined by its investment with libido, regardless of any positive or negative affective value.[1] By insisting that the loss that precedes the work of mourning is not necessarily a loss of a person loved by the subject, Lacan attempts to emphasize that the object of mourning is not determined by the subject's affective attitude, but rather by another "special function" that this object holds in the subject's libidinal economy. This is one of Lacan's major contributions to Freud's theory of mourning: the characterization of this special function as being a placeholder for the subject's own fantasized desirability. In other words, the person lost and then mourned is not necessarily a person whom the subject loves, it is a person who is considered to love the subject; that is, it is a person who holds a special part in their heart *for* the subject as desired or, in other words, functions as the cause of its desire (p. 117).

At this point, it is useful to address Lacan's distinction between the object cause of desire (also called *objet petit a* and, from now on the object *a*) and the object of desire. The object of desire is the object towards which desire tends.

Desire works in such a way that, whenever we get our hands on the object we desire, desire withers for a moment only to re-emerge as a desire for another object. In this sense, one should talk of objects of desire in the plural: a chain of objects whose common denominator is subjective. The object *a* is the algebraic notation of the common denominator of the subject's desirous tendencies. It is what *causes* desire rather than the object towards which it intends. It sets desire in motion and is said to define the conditions that determine the features that make specific objects desirable for the subject. Being a condition for desire rather than an object desired, the object *a* is not conceived as a positivistic object that materializes in reality. The object *a* is better described as a placeholder: a constitutive site of a lack that keeps desire searching for some object to fill it up with.

Absence can only appear within presence and *vice versa* (Lacan, 2006, p. 497). More precisely, Lacan argues that "lack is only graspable through the intermediary of the symbolic" (Lacan, 2014, p. 132). He gives a compelling example when he states that, when visiting a library, one can only notice that a volume is missing when a system of symbolic indexing was previously put in place. In the same way, the object *a* can only be designated as a lack when it is situated in the symbolic. And, conversely, because the object *a* is in itself a lack, it functions as the background on which the symbolic designation of the object of desire is inscribed.

Lacan argues that there is a structural homology in the work of mourning and the psychotic process (Lacan, 2019, p. 336, 347). First of all, he states that they both entail a "foreclosure" (*forclusion*) (Lacan, 1997, p. 321). Foreclosure is a psychic mechanism that is situated at the origin of psychosis. Basically, foreclosure operates by radically rejecting a particular signifier from the symbolic order (p. 15). In the case of psychosis, this is a primordial signifier that Lacan calls the Name-of-the-Father (p. 96).[2] This primordial signifier is constitutively repressed and plays a crucial role in the establishment of the symbolic order. Describing foreclosure in spatial terms, Lacan argues that it creates a "hole in the symbolic" in the place where this primordial signifier is inscribed in the unconscious (p. 156). Therefore, one could say that foreclosure creates a hole in the place of a lack in the symbolic. Lacan clearly distinguishes the status of a hole and a lack. While a lack is considered to be a symbolic designation of an absence, a hole implies the disappearance of the symbolic order, representing an effect of the real. This is why, according to Lacan, other terms can be inscribed on the background of lack, while the hole allows no such inscription to take place.

Lacan argues that the loss that precedes mourning can be associated with a foreclosure that introduces a hole in the symbolic (Lacan, 2019, p. 336). Namely, the intolerable experience of the death of a "special someone" for the subject is translated in spatial terms as a creation of a hole in the symbolic in the place of the object *a*. This is the *initiatory aspect* of the work of mourning. The *compensatory aspect* of the work of mourning is the successive attempt to patch up the hole created in reality. It involves an attempt to clarify something in relation to this hole, in as much as it is situated in the place of the object *a* (pp. 337, 345–346). The compensatory aspect of mourning is homologous to the work of delusions in cases of psychosis; however, there are some crucial differences. Psychotic delusions come to compensate for the foreclosure of a central organizing signifier from the symbolic order (the Name-of-the-Father). In this sense, they come to compensate for a fundamental symbolic destabilization that puts the consistency of the symbolic as a whole at risk. The work of mourning is done in order to compensate for the temporary loss of the site of lack (the object *a*) in the symbolic. Lacan is explicitly suspicious of psychoanalysts who view delusions as a cure for psychosis. He carefully employs terms such as "stabilization" (Lacan, 1997, pp. 69, 86, 140) in order to describe the best possible outcome achieved through the delusional reconstruction of symbolic reality in psychosis. On the other hand, the work of mourning, when it comes to an end, provides a valid substitute for the site of lack in the symbolic. One could say that this is due to the fact that, while in psychosis, the subject attempts to mend an irremediable hole created in the place of the Name-of-the-Father; in mourning, the symbolic labor is done with the aim of redefining the circumference of the site of a lack. Thus, one could argue that, in order to gain back one's desire and be able to invest it in other objects, in mourning, one reworks the circumference of the object *a* in the symbolic. Lacan adds that the subject does so by "authenticating" the reality of the preceding loss "little by little, piece by piece, sign by sign" (Lacan, 2017B, p. 396). These signs are the imaginary and symbolic attributes of the love object.

In order to better understand the effect of the work of mourning on the circumference of the object *a*, a paragraph from Lacan's *Seminar X: Anxiety (1962-1963)* is worth considering:

> As for us, the work of mourning strikes us, in a light that is at once identical and contrary, as a labour that is carried out to maintain and sustain all these painstaking links with the aim of restoring the bond with the true object of relation, the masked object, the object *a*—for which thereafter a substitute can be given that will ultimately have no more scope than the one that initially occupied this place ... The problem of mourning is the problem of maintaining ... the bonds whereby desire is suspended, not from the object *a*, but from *i(a)*.
>
> (Lacan, 2014, p. 335)

In this paragraph, we see that Lacan argues that, in mourning, the subject does not engage with the elaboration of the object *a* itself, but with the idealized dimension that narcissistically structures all love relationships: the image of the object *a*—commonly notated as *i(a)*—associated by Lacan with the ideal ego.

The ideal ego is one of the prototypical psychic components constituting the Freudian ego. In his account of the mirror stage, Lacan describes the ideal ego as the most "primordial form" of ego construction prior to its functioning in the formation of self-identity and the establishment of intersubjective relations (Lacan, 2006, p. 76). It functions as an *imaginary* ideal of perfection that masks the fragmented reality of the infant's body. It embodies the illusion, fascination, and seduction that is particularly associated with the relationship between the ego and the specular image. In the developed model of the mirror stage, where Lacan attempts to incorporate the function of the object *a*, the ideal ego is represented by the formula: *i(a)*. This formula stands for the series of images of the object *a* in as far as they are represented in the narcissistic "misrecognition" taking place in the mirror stage. The *i(a)* stands for the imaginary totality of the ego that is associated with the way in which the subject is viewed by the Other (Lacan, 2014, p. 40). More precisely, the ideal ego embodies the idealized imaginary traits that make the subject desirable in the eyes of the Other; namely, that makes the subject the object of the Other's desire.

Lacan emphasizes that the object *a* can only be pursued as masked behind the veil of the image (Lacan, 2019, p. 373). Thus, the work of mourning is now better understood as the progressive re-signification of the subject as desirable on the imaginary level of the *i(a)* (Lacan, 2019, p. 347).

We can now see that the identification with the lost object is not reserved for melancholia but is essential in mourning as well (Lacan, 2014, p. 111). In mourning, the subject identifies with the lost object in order to regain access to its own narcissistic image reflected from the mirror situated in the place of the Other (Lacan, 2017A, p. 287; 2014, p. 141). Tragically, this means that, when Laertes leaps into Ophelia's grave to hold her once again in his arms, he is mourning not her but the loss of his narcissistic image reflected in her eyes.

As soon as the subject's narcissistic image is re-established in the symbolic, a place for a lack that would kick start desire is created. This can also create a shift in one's mode of desiring and in the characteristics of the objects of desire. This shift might be minimal or drastic and, can be referred to as being creative, as will be described in the next sections. This brings the work of mourning to an end and lets the subject continue on with their life.

On the side of melancholia, Lacan argues that we are dealing with a different type of object, one that is "much harder to get a handle on" (Lacan, 2017B, p. 396). He adds that, in comparison to the object of mourning, the object of melancholia is "thoroughly veiled, masked, and obscure," lacking any trait that the subject could rework or authenticate through the work of mourning (p. 396). This veiled object is the object *a* itself.

As mentioned earlier, the object *a* is not like any object of exchange. It is an object that is originally and constitutively lacking. One could say that the object *a* is itself equivalent to a lack in the unconscious. Being a site of an unattainable absence, it functions as the *cause* of desire, propping desire in its perpetual trajectory. Lacan emphasizes that "not all of the libidinal investment passes by way of the specular image" (Lacan, 2014, p 38). Therefore, when described in relation to *i(a),* he explicitly argues that the object *a* "is this remainder, this residue, this object whose status escapes the status of the object derived from the specular image" (p. 40).

Lacan argues that, in the work of melancholia, the subject does not suffice with the circumference of the object *a*—the re-signification of the ideal ego, the *i(a)*—but aims to achieve a "radical reference to the *a*" (p. 336). In doing so, the melancholic "initially … attacks this image so as to reach, within it, the object *a* that transcends him … [an object that is] fundamentally misrecognized and alienated in the narcissistic relation" (pp. 335–336; brackets added).

Thus, we see that, while mourning identification directs the work to the level of the *i(a)*, melancholia is characterized by a "more mysterious" form of narcissistic identification with the object *a* itself (Lacan, 2017A, p. 283; 2014, p. 37). However, without the veil of the image, the object *a* lacks consistency and is impossible to identify with (Lacan, 2019, p. 373). This impossibility brings about the debasement of the ego on the level of the ego-ideal. The ego-ideal (also referred to as *I*) is another crucial prototypical aspect of the ego (Lacan, 1988, pp. 125–126). Unlike the ideal ego—which represents an idealized image that the subject sees as itself—the ego-ideal represents the symbolic vantage point from which the subject perceives itself as it is seen by others or the vantage point from where the subject gains its position in society (Vanheule, 2011, p. 4). Lacan argues that the threat of the ego-ideal when confronted by the object *a* can only be mitigated through the "defense" of the ideal ego (Lacan, 2017B, p. 394). This is why, when turning away from the ideal ego the subject also forfeits its access to the ego-ideal. Therefore, the identification with the object *a* in melancholia unravels a subjective position in which the ego, in both of its prototypical aspects, is insufficient in filling the constitutive absence of the object *a* (Lacan, 2017A, p. 282). In other words, for the melancholic, nothing about the "self" can be a good enough reason to put an end to the overwhelming desolation opened by the narcissistic identification with the constitutive absence of the object *a*.

Slavoj Žižek (2000) argues that melancholic identification entails the disavowal of the fact that the object *a* "is lacking from the very beginning, that its emergence coincides with its lack, that this object is nothing but the positivization of a void or lack, a purely anamorphic entity that does not exist in itself" (p. 660). Through the unconditional fixation on the object *a*, the melancholic expresses a yearning for an absolute reality beyond ordinary reality—beyond the imaginary or the symbolic. Thus, melancholia is not so much characterized by a desire that lost its object but by a world of desired objects deprived of the reason to desire them. It entails a movement from loss to lack (p. 659), from the *i(a)* to the *a*; a movement that can also be described as a movement from the imaginary and the symbolic to the real as the rootstock of identification.

Žižek adds that by aiming beyond the imaginary idealized image and remaining faithful to the object *a*, the work of melancholia gains a level of "conceptual and ethical primacy" (p. 658). Instead of aiming at the particular characteristics of *i(a)*, it takes the subject to the *limits* of the universal; a gesture that Lacan associated with Kantian ethics that, at their limit, bring the subject to accept its own death in the name of the so-called categorical imperative (Lacan, 1992, 189). Kant defines the categorical imperative as a universal moral law that one must follow, regardless of their desires or personal well-being. On the same note, the work of melancholia disregards the welfare of the subject with the aim of achieving something on the level of the absolute.

This self-destructive identificatory gesture brings about a form of "remorse" that involves "something along the lines of suicide on the part of the object" (Lacan, 2017B, p. 397). Lacan relates this to an attempt to drag the object to a "suicide-rush," making a leap right through the imaginary montage of the ideal ego into a place of lack, where the symbolic provides no support, just like jumping through a window (Lacan, 2014, pp. 335–336). Due to the identification with the object *a*, the suicide of the object is directly tied to the death of the ego itself (Lacan, 2017A, p. 283).

Lacan argues that *i(a)* and the object *a* are the pillars of the function of desire (Lacan, 2014, p. 41). Accordingly, by foregoing the *i(a)* and through the suicide of the object *a*, the subject is compelled to turn away from desire as a whole. This is why Lacan argues that melancholia is a form of pathological mourning that "triggers infinitely more catastrophic effects" (Lacan, 2017B, p. 396); these are effects that hinder what Freud (1917) described as "the instinct [*Triebes*] which compels every living thing to cling to life" (p. 246).

Creativity in Lacan

Lacan was very much interested in the domain of artistic creativity. He was an avid reader and consumer of the arts. As a young psychiatrist, he was known to mingle with creative writers, attending group readings along with notable figures at the famous Parisian bookstore, *Shakespeare & Co.* (Roudinesco, 1997, pp. 12–13). Lacan is also particularly known to be influenced by the surrealist movement in France, mingling with the likes of André Breton and René Crevel (p. 18). Surrealism—an artistic movement that was influenced by Freud from its very inception—was very much interested in the notion of the unconscious, which dictated that creativity itself be considered a liberation from the control of reason. Lacan was not only personally interested in the creative domain, but his encounter with the art world also greatly affected his psychoanalytic teaching. His allusions to ancient and classical paintings, his reflections on famous books and plays, and his engagement with musical pieces accompanied the whole of his teaching and took a major role in his unique conceptualizations.

In his seventh seminar, Lacan (1992) devotes a whole session—entitled "On Creation *ex nihilo*"—to the theme of creativity. In this session, Lacan presents a secularized notion of creativity, secularized not only in a theological sense but also in the sense that it is neither romantic nor humanistic. Simply put, for Lacan, the power of creativity resides neither in God nor in the autonomous subject but rather in the signifier itself (Chaitin, 1996, pp. 64–65). For Lacan, reality itself, and anything that could potentially be included in it, rests on the signifier: "the reality with which we are concerned is upheld, woven through, constituted, by a tress of signifiers" (Lacan, 1997, p. 249). It is with no exception that he argues that, in terms of creativity, "as far as the signifier is concerned …

man is the artisan of his support system" (Lacan, 1992, p. 119). In other words, human creativity can only be expressed through signifiers and on the basis of their capacity for signification.

In the same session, Lacan describes the creative act as an attempt to elevate an ordinary object to a "dignity" that it did not possess before (p. 118). He associates this act with Freud's account of sublimation: a process in which libidinal energies are channeled from strictly sexual objects into socially valued objects such as those created in the arts (Freud, 1905, pp. 178–179). In other words, sublimation entails changing the object and its aim. First, the object is de-sexualized. Second, its new aim, while being "closely related" to the previous one, is raised to a higher level that is "free from objection" and "more socially valuable" (Freud, 1910, pp. 15, 29). Lacan goes beyond Freud when he argues that sublimation does not necessarily entail a change of objects but involves adjusting the position of the object in the symbolic. More precisely, Lacan argues that sublimation strives to raise an object "to the dignity of the Thing" (Lacan, 1992, p. 112).

Lacan's account of the Thing (*das Ding*) is based on the distinction between two German words: *die Sache* ("Things") and *das Ding*. "Things," according to Lacan, are object-representations as they manifest in the symbolic order. He associates them with what Freud called "thing-representations" (1915, p. 203), which, in German, are called "*Sachvorstellungen.*" Lacan argues that Freud refers to "The Thing" as an object beyond representation (e.g., Freud, 1894, p. 62). He associated it with what is impossible to know (Lacan, 1992, p. 55), with a thing in the "beyond-of-the-signified" (p. 54), "characterized by the fact that it is impossible for us to imagine it" (p. 125). He adds that it occupies the place of a primordial psychic constituent that Freud identified as being beyond the pleasure principle and that Lacan refers to as the "primordial real" (p. 118).

The distinction between symbolic representation and the beyond-of-the-signified is analogous to Lacan's distinction between symbolic "reality" and the "real." Reality is that which is constituted via signifiers—what is upheld, woven through, and constituted, by signifiers in the symbolic order (Lacan, 1997, p. 249). However, the symbolic order is not a totality (p. 183). For Lacan, the symbolic is not whole as it is always lacking and incomplete. This is what Lacan describes as the *lack in the Other* (Lacan, 2017A, p. 373), which on other occasions is expressed in the contention that "there is no Other of the Other" (Lacan, 2006, p. 688). In some instances of his teaching, the real is identified by Lacan as this mode of symbolic incompleteness, as the name of what is impossible to articulate in its totality within the symbolic. It is what is outside the field of representation and resists signification, thus making the gap between reality and the real unbridgeable.

Lacan stresses that, when sublimation aims to elevate an object to the "dignity" of the Thing, it can never truly transform the object to the Thing-in-itself (i.e., the primordial real), because sublimation is, in itself, an act of signification (Lacan, 1992, p. 118).[3] The Thing-in-itself is beyond representation; it is sublime, in as much as it can only function as a "regulative principle" for sublimation: in

Kantian terms, a principle that guides a certain practice but remains unreachable by itself (Kant, 1998, pp. 297–298 [A179/B222]). Sublimation then can only be said to follow the path of the sublime but never to reach it; that is, never to produce something of the real in reality. Therein lies what Lacan calls the "problem of sublimation" (Lacan, 1992, p. 125) and, for the sake of our discussion, the problem of creativity as well: they are both confined to the disjunction between the symbolic and the real and, therefore, can only fashion the object in the image of the Thing that is impossible to imagine.

This is why, for Lacan, creativity and alienation are two sides of the same coin (Stavrakakis, 2007, p. 48). Any creative act attempts to capture something that is unimaginable prior to the act of creation, something beyond-the-signified. However, because the symbolic order is inherently lacking, any object of creation will never be able to truly embody the primordial real. It could only provide a supplement, one which might have immense cultural value but still will not be able to bridge the gap between the symbolic and the real. This inherent limitation of the symbolic dictates the alienating dimension of any form of creation and prevents the creative act from realizing the romantic fantasy of infinite creativity.

However, while the lack in the Other functions as a limit to creativity, it is also the condition that enables Lacan's psychoanalysis to transgress the confines of strict structuralism and leave room for the emergence of desire. For Lacan, lack is always related to desire. Specifically, lack is the cause of desire (Lacan, 2017B, p. 139). This notion has already been explicated in terms of the object a in the previous section. When described in terms of the lack in the Other, the desire of the Other is determined as the thing that the Other is lacking and wants to have. When saying that "man's desire is the desire of the Other" (Lacan, 2001, p. 235), Lacan is insinuating that desire is first engendered when one asks *what does the Other want that is beyond me?* The answers to this question come in the form of signifiers and images that determine the idealized traits that make one desirable in the eyes of the Other. It is by identifying with these traits that the subject's desire receives its specific features and is set in motion.

Therefore, we see that the lack in the Other plays two roles in the creative act. On the one hand, it limits the work of sublimation and alienates the creative act. On the other hand, it is the condition for the establishment of the desire to create, keeping desire going in its perpetual attempt to capture the uncapturable or represent the unrepresentable. In other words, it is what keeps desire metonymically sliding on the chain of signifiers, circumventing the confines of its indiscernible cause.

The twofold function of the lack in the Other stems from what Lacan characterizes as the unique *extimate* relationship between the symbolic and the real (Lacan, 1992, p. 139).[4] From a Lacanian perspective, the real resists symbolization but also persists alongside the symbolic. One can venture to say that it affects the symbolic through the continuous resurgence of negativity, a negativity that limits the inventive outlook of the creative subject. Therefore, it is the persistence and irreducibility of the Real that deflects the limits of human creativity and thus enables the moment of creation. In this moment, the lack in the Other is dislocated, making way for a singular symbolic fabrication that is accompanied by a certain satisfaction that allows creative desire to move towards the next object.

Creativity in mourning and melancholia

Philosopher Giorgio Agamben presents a unique and inventive reformulation of the Freudian analysis of mourning and melancholia in his book *Stanzas* (1993). Agamben endorses the Freudian economic characterization of melancholia as well as its comparability with the process of mourning. However, he proposes a different characterization for its point of origin, one which allows him to offer a new theory of creativity. Agamben emphasizes Freud's argument that, in contrast to mourning, it is difficult to identify the point of origin where the initial loss of an object prompts the onset of melancholia. Agamben adds, in contrast to Freud, that the lost object is not only indiscernible to consciousness but, in fact, there is no possibility of pinpointing the actuality of the lost melancholic object at all. This is because the initiatory aspect of melancholia is not a loss but the inward withdrawal of libidinal energy itself, while the origin of the process of mourning is an actual loss of a love object. Accordingly, Agamben characterizes melancholia as a unique and separate form of mourning, devoid of an actual lost object: a unique form of mourning that is "an intention to mourn that precedes and anticipates the loss of the object" (p. 20). He defines melancholia as a spontaneous attempt to reallocate a large sum of libidinal energy in an endeavor that revolves around a non-existent object. In this endeavor, the libido functions as though a loss has occurred, even though such a loss has never occurred.

Up to this point, Agamben remains within the scope of the Lacanian description of mourning and melancholia. He adds his original interpretation when he argues—in opposition to Freud—that melancholia is *not* a pathological form of mourning; that is, it should not be considered an inappropriate regressive response to the loss of a love object, but rather a unique *creative process* that aims to transform an unobtainable unknown object into a lost object. Going beyond Ernst Kris' (1936/1952) characterization of artistic creativity as a "regression in the service of the ego" (p. 177), Agamben argues that melancholia "would be not so much the regressive reaction to the loss of the love object as the imaginative capacity to make an unobtainable object appear as if lost" (Agamben, 1993, p. 20). In other words, rather than defining melancholia in terms of regression, Agamben defines melancholia as an ambitious creative process that aims to transform what was never in existence into a retrospectively obtainable lost object. Agamben claims that the work of melancholia is essentially characterized by this radically creative strategy. It is a process that seeks to engender a space for the existence of the non-existent by the creative construction of a mental scene (the melancholic scene) in which what could have only been an object of thought and imagination gains a "phantasmagorical reality" as an object that has been lost and is now mourned (p. 20).

Armed with a better understanding of Lacan's view on creativity and with Agamben's interpretation of melancholia, we are now ready to reassess the question of mourning and melancholia as creative endeavors. So let us go on and try to imagine both the mourner and the melancholic as artists who are engaging in a creative act and let us attempt to distinguish the two when they are conceived in this way.

In the past, the work of mourning has been associated with the work of sublimation, in as much as both processes revolve around the symbolization of an unreachable object (Roussillon, 2005; Civitarese, 2016). The "object-representations" taking part in mourning are the signifiers and images that convey the idealized attributes of the subject as desirable for the Other. In the work of mourning, these attributes are raised to the "dignity" of the object *a*. In other words, they mark out a site in the symbolic for the subject as desiring—for the cause of desire. This brings the work of mourning to an end and, in terms of sublimation, adjusts the position of the subject in the symbolic, granting it access to the social domain. It is by submitting to dependency on the symbolic—i.e., by finding the site for libidinal re-investment in the signifier—that the subject is liberated from its dependence on the foreclosed object and overcomes the hole situated in its place in the symbolic (Kristeva, 2005, p. 1660). Thus, we see that the work of mourning directly depends on the creative use of language that is dependent on the signifier. Both the mourner and the artist engage in the symbolic re-articulation of the boundaries of fantasy or, put differently, of the subject's imaginary relationship with the specular image. Therefore, when we say that the mourner and the artist express something singular in their work, we argue that they give symbolic form to that which they are able to extract from their particular identifications with the ideal image that they associate with the Thing.

This mode of creativity can bring about a change in the position of the subject. This change is the end result of the persistent resurfacing of a traumatic real at the threshold of the symbolic, a real that uncovers a lack in the discursive structure and stimulates the desire for a new articulation. Thus, what is created in the work of mourning is always related to the emergence of new signifiers that organize the relationship between the subject and the Other. These can be either signifiers that demarcate a site of "remembering" (Lacan, 2006, p. 521)[5] or master signifiers that function as a "quilting point" (*point de capiton*). Briefly put, the "quilting point" is a concept that originates in Lacan's work on psychosis (Lacan, 1997, pp. 258–270). It is used to describe a symbolic operation in which a master signifier serves as an "anchoring point" that organizes the chain of signifiers as a whole. Accordingly, mourning can also be determined as a rejuvenating process after which the subject's position in the symbolic order dramatically changes. This sheds new light on the famous saying: "Tis better to have loved and lost than never to have loved at all." However, from a Lacanian perspective, we might say: "Tis better to have *been* loved and lose *the one who loved you*," as the work of mourning can radically reshape one's way of loving or, better yet, of desiring.

Melancholia can also be referred to as a form of sublimation. In his paper, "The Ego and the Id" (1923), Freud describes a "negative" form of sublimation that sheds light on the relationship between sublimation and melancholia and is worth being quoted at length:

> Through its work of identification and sublimation it [the ego] gives the death instincts [*Todestrieben*] in the id assistance in gaining control over the libido, but in so doing it runs the risk of becoming the object of the death instincts [*Todestrieben*] and of itself perishing. In order to be able to help in this way it has had itself to become filled with libido; it thus itself becomes the representative of Eros and thenceforward desires to live and to be loved. But since the ego's work of sublimation results in a diffusion of the instincts [*Triebentmischung*] and a liberation of the aggressive instincts [*Aggressionstriebe*] in the super-ego, its struggle against the libido exposes it to the danger of maltreatment and death.
>
> (Freud, 1923, p. 56; brackets added)[6]

This passage is extremely interesting, as it describes a process of sublimation in which the ego runs the risk of becoming the object of the death drive (*Todestrieben*) and thus perishing. We see that sublimation can either be "positive" and divert the drive to higher grounds where the superego can elevate its work to the level of a socially valued activity, or it can become "negative" and direct the drive inwards and cause the death of the ego. The latter demonstrates the foreboding and destructive aspect of sublimation that betrays its reliance on the symbolic. It is what happens when sublimation becomes "excessive" and directs the subject towards an impossible ideal based on an overvaluation of the lost object. It is my hypothesis that this form of excessive sublimation can be associated with the unique type of creativity that takes place in melancholia.

The melancholic senses that human reality, social norms, and values are all dependent on objects of identification that are symbolically predetermined. This predetermination is accurately assessed by the melancholic as exemplifying the "stupid" dimension of the signifier, culminating in the fact that all these modes of identification are alienated (Lacan, 1998, pp. 19–21). In his creative endeavor, the melancholic is determined to *refuse* the alienating dimension of the signifier. This position is radical as it aims to create some*Thing* beyond the realm of *thing-representation*. It entails what Freud describes as the loss of cathexis in the out-side world, seen in psychosis. In terms borrowed from Lacan, we might say that, due to the fixation on *the Thing*, the melancholic position entails losing interest in the *things* that constitute reality.

Freud (1914) describes the loss of cathexis in the outside world as a second-ary pathological form of narcissistic regression (pp. 74–75, 84). Correspondingly, when losing interest in symbolic reality, the melancholic diverts his creative resources to the ego. Thus, while the creative work of mourning materializes in the interstice of the imaginary and the symbolic, the melancholic process materializes on the threshold of the real (object *a*). Viewed in this way, melancholic creativity is not considered to raise object-representations to the "dignity" of the Thing but, through a problematic mode of identification, to attempt to raise the ego to the "dignity" of an indiscernible fantasized ideal that is based on the overvaluation of the object *a*. This is a transition from a creation that revolves around lack, to a process of creation *in excess*—as according to Lacan, "there is no absence in the real" (Lacan, 1991, p. 313).

The melancholic excessive creative outlook involves a leap of faith that disavows the *extimate* relationship between the symbolic and the Real. More specifically, what is perceived as the "internal" is split between a used-up reproachable ego and a phantasmagorical "primordial" and "pre-symbolic" ego that is identified with the overevaluated and indiscernible ideal of the object *a*. This phantasmagorical ego becomes the source of the melancholic creative drive. It operates as a principally unrepresentable point of reference that functions as an impossible cause of desire in the creative act. This narcissistic mode of operation is aimed at creating an object that is totally enclosed in itself: a fantasy of a lasting existence of an idiosyncratic ego, independent from the symbolic domain. In this sense, it can be described as a truly essentialist endeavor that disavows the fundamental alienation that structures subjectivity and the fact that desire and creation are marked by an irreducible gap. By disavowing this gap and attempting to force a continuity between the primordial real and the place of the phantasmagorical primordial ego, the melancholic sets on an impossible creative process that disregards the dialectics of desire as they are described by Lacan. This is a creative process that dismisses the limits of human creativity and egoic autonomy. This contradictory position conditions the melancholic scene: a scene that aims to guarantee at all costs the prospects of the non-alienated phantasmagorical reality of an idiosyncratic "pre-symbolic" ego, ignoring its dire implications for one's reality.

In this sense, one can describe the melancholic as the creative artist *par-excellence*: a creator endowed with an "ethical primacy" in the field of creation (Žižek, 2000, p. 658). However, this excessive form of creativity comes at a cost. While, in mourning, the subject is able to take the lead and bring the process to an end, "in melancholia, this process clearly doesn't come to a conclusion because the object takes the helm. The object triumphs" (Lacan, 2014, p. 335).

In conclusion, it is the particularity of the identificatory relationships with the object that distinguishes mourning and melancholia as two creative processes. In mourning, the creative work revolves around the *i(a)*: an object that is inscribed on the side of the Other. For the melancholic, the creative work revolves around the object *a*; however, this object is situated on the side of the subject and identified with a phantasmagorical idiosyncratic "pre-symbolic" ego. The former can be considered a "transitive" creative process because it aims at an object in reality. The latter can be defined as an "intransitive" and "excessive" creative process, as its object is inherently lacking, and the process never comes to an end (Brenner, 2019).

Creativity in the treatment of melancholia

In *Seminar VII: The Ethics of Psychoanalysis (1959–1960)* Lacan claims that it seems there is indeed something in common between creative artistic enthusiasm and the onset of melancholia (Lacan, 1992, pp. 116–117). In this chapter, I provided support for this claim and suggested that melancholia be described as an excessive creative process, which exhausts one's capacity to desire and breaks one's ties with reality. However, in agreement with Agamben (1993), I would like to suggest that the relationship between creativity and melancholia should not necessarily be understood as a strictly pathological one. It might be the case that a meta-psychological framework that explicates a unique type of excessive melancholic creativity can be useful in developing further psychoanalytic interventions for the treatment of melancholia.

Creativity and creative tasks have been used in the treatment of major depression for many years, chiefly in the fields of art therapy (Reynolds, 2000; Gussak, 2007) and occupational therapy (Griffiths, 2008; Hees *et al.*, 2010). Practitioners are known to suggest that creative tasks facilitate learning and problem-solving skills; deepen a patient's capacity for introspection and emotional self-awareness; provide patients with a sense of satisfaction and self-esteem; and contribute to a patient's feeling of self-worth by getting acknowledgement from their peers. All of these contribute to a patient's sense of having their life under control and supposedly help with the treatment of major depression.

From a Lacanian perspective, I have so far attributed the problem of melancholia to an excessive form of creativity that is conditioned by the over-evaluation of the object *a*. The traits of the object *a*—being in itself thoroughly veiled, masked, and obscure—cannot be seen or truly investigated by the subject. Therefore, the melancholic remains defenseless against the destructive force of the impossible elaboration of this object in the creative process.

When discussing the psychoanalytic treatment of melancholia, Lacan (2017B) stresses that the subject's complaint does not materialize on the level of the ideal ego, as "the melancholic never tells you that he looks bad, that his face is at its worst, or that it is contorted" (p. 396). Lacan argues that the complaint materializes on the level of the ego-ideal, when the melancholic "tells you that he is the lowest of the low, that he brings on one catastrophe after another for his entire family, and so on" (p. 396). This emphasizes the problematic the melancholic faces in establishing a symbolic supplement to the real of the object *a*.

Accordingly, Lacan adds that the work with melancholics is work on the "limit" between the symbolic and the real. In this work, he says, "we must know how to get the subject to stay away from this limit" (p. 397). Specifically, he says that psychoanalysts have to be attentive to the function of the signifier in as much as it establishes the position of the ego-ideal only in a "roundabout manner" (p. 397), i.e., through the imaginary identification on the level of the ideal ego, with the *i(a)*. In other words, because the threat of the ego-ideal when confronted by the object *a* can only be mitigated through the "defense" of the ideal ego (p. 394), the treatment of melancholia can be said to revolve around the mobilization of the dynamic qualities of the *i(a)* in the imaginary, which can function as a limit to the hold of the object *a* on the *I*.

Taking after Lacan in his seminar on Joyce (2016), one might argue that the work with melancholic subjects revolves around the construction of the "*escabeau*" (p. 145). Directly translated as "stepladder," the *escabeau* is a small step that the subject can use to raise itself to the level of the Beautiful (*Beau*). As Miller (2016) argues, the *escabeau* is a product of a unique type of a "Freudian sublimation, but in its intersection with narcissism" (p. 7). Therefore, we describe it as a construction on the level of the signified rather than the signifier—the imaginary rather than the symbolic. Particularly in the context of this chapter, we describe it as a construct that materializes when the subject raises something of the ideal ego to the level of the grand ideals of the Good, the True, and the Beautiful. Accordingly, Miller adds that "creators of *escabeaus* ... are designed to make art with the symptom, with the opaque *jouissance* of the symptom" (p. 7). In doing so, they produce beauty from their narcissistic ideals, which function as "the last defense against the real" (p. 7).

Correspondingly, in the case of melancholic subjects, one might argue that psychoanalytic work strives to harness their creative efforts to construct an *escabeau* that would function as a defense against the real of the object *a*. In contrast to the treatment of neurosis, which comes to elaborate the singularity of one's suffering beyond imaginary identifications on the level of the *i(a)*, the treatment of melancholia aims to universalize the *i(a)* in the creation of the Beautiful. In practical terms, this means directing the psychoanalytic treatment towards the exploration of the subject's narcissistic interests and their creative incorporation in fields such as ethics (e.g., of work), aesthetics of the body (e.g., in sports), and art, harnessing the subject's uncompromising diligence for the creation of an object of beauty. Following Lacan (2017B), this work would entail identifying the traits of the *i(a)* *via* the melancholic's criticism of the *I*. Lacan states that being attentive to these criticisms can "help put us on the scent" (p. 396) and aid psychoanalysts in facilitating the administration of the subject's creativity on the level of the *i(a)* or, stated otherwise, in diverting the focus of the treatment from the excessive sublimation on the threshold of the symbolic and real to working out the traits of the *i(a)* in the imaginary so that they could function as the rootstock for the construction of the *escabeau*.

Notes

1 Not to mention the fact that Freud describes love and hate as two sides of the same coin (Freud, 1909, p. 134).
2 See an extensive account of psychotic foreclosure in Brenner, 2020, pp. 63–100.
3 In his description of *das Ding* in seminar VII, Lacan is alluding to Kant's notion of the "thing-in-itself." See Kant, 1998.
4 Lacan coins the term *extimacy* (*extimité*) by applying the prefix *ex* from *exterieur* to the word *intimité*. The resulting neologism expresses the way in which the opposition

between the symbolic and the real cannot be strictly perceived as an "inside" and "outside" but as an "intimate exteriority" (Lacan, 1992, p. 139).

5 As Lacan says in "The Direction of the Treatment and the Principles of its Power": "one does not get better because one remembers. One remembers because one gets better." (2006, p. 521)

6 Notice that I've added the original German for "death instincts," "diffusion of instincts" and "aggressive instincts." All of these have been wrongly translated as having to do with the instincts instead of the drives. In the body of this chapter I will address them as drives.

References

Agamben, G. (1993) *Stanzas: Word and Phantasm in Western Culture*. Minneapolis: University of Minnesota Press.

American Psychiatric Association. (2013) *Diagnostic and Statistical Manual of Mental Disorders* (5th ed.). https://doi.org/10.1176/appi.books.9780890425596

Aristotle, E. W. D. R. (1927) *Problemata*. Oxford: Clarendon Press.

Brenner, L. S. (2019) 'Creative Hyper-Activation in Depression', *Creativity Research Journal*, 31(4), pp. 359–370.

Bulloch, A., Williams, J., Lavorato, D., & Patten, S. (2014) 'Recurrence of Major Depressive Episodes is Strongly Dependent on the Number of Previous Episodes,' *Depression and Anxiety*, *31*(1), pp. 72–76.

Carhart-Harris, R. L., Mayberg, H. S., Malizia, A. L., & Nutt, D. (2008) 'Mourning and Melancholia Revisited: Correspondences between Principles of Freudian Metapsychology and Empirical Findings in Neuropsychiatry', *Annals of General Psychiatry*, 7, p. 9. https://doi.org/10.1186/1744-859X-7-9

Chaitin, G. D. (1996) *Rhetoric and Culture in Lacan*. Cambridge, UK: Cambridge University Press.

Chávez-Eakle, R. A., Lara, M. del C., & Cruz-Fuentes, C. (2006) 'Personality: A Possible Bridge between Creativity and Psychopathology? *Creativity Research Journal*, *18*(1), pp. 27–38.

Chruszczewski, M. H. (2014) 'The Creative Side of Mood Disorders', *Creativity*, 1, pp. 46–64.

Civitarese, G. (2016) 'On Sublimation', *The International Journal of Psychoanalysis*, 97, pp. 1369–1392.

Corazza, G. E. (2016) 'Potential Originality and Effectiveness: The Dynamic Definition of Creativity', *Creativity Research Journal*, 28, pp. 258–267.

Frantom, C., & Sherman, M. F. (1999) 'At what Price Art? Affective Instability within a Visual Art Population', *Creativity Research Journal*, *12*(1), pp. 15–23.

Freud, S. (1894) 'Die Abwehr-Neuropsychosen', *Gesammelte Were*, 1, pp. 59–74.

Freud, S. (1905) 'Three Essays on the Theory of Sexuality', in J. Strachey (Ed.), *The Standard Edition of the Complete Psychological Works of Sigmund Freud*, Volume 7. London: The Hogarth Press and the Institute of Psycho-Analysis, pp. 123–246.

Freud, S. (1909) 'Analysis of a Phobia in a Five-Year-Old Boy', in J. Strachey (Ed.), *The Standard Edition of the Complete Psychological Works of Sigmund Freud*, Volume 10. London: The Hogarth Press and the Institute of Psycho-Analysis, pp. 1–150.

Freud, S. (1910) 'The Origin and Development of Psychoanalysis', *American Journal of Psychology*, 21(2), pp. 181–218.

Freud, S. (1914) 'On Narcissism', in J. Strachey (Ed.), *The Standard Edition of the Complete Psychological Works of Sigmund Freud*, Volume 14. London: The Hogarth Press and the Institute of Psycho-Analysis, pp. 67–102.

Freud, S. (1915) 'The Unconscious', in J. Strachey (Ed.), *The Standard Edition of the Complete Psychological Works of Sigmund Freud*, Volume 14. London: The Hogarth Press and the Institute of Psycho-Analysis, pp. 159–215.

Griffiths, S. (2008) 'The Experience of Creative Activity as a Treatment Medium', *Journal of Mental Health*, 17, pp. 49–63.

Gussak, D. (2007) 'The Effectiveness of Art Therapy in Reducing Depression in Prison Populations', *International Journal of Offender Therapy and Comparative Criminology*, 51, pp. 444–460.

Hees, H. L., Koeter, M. W. J., de Vries, G., Ooteman, W., & Schene, A. H. (2010) 'Effectiveness of Adjuvant Occupational Therapy in Employees with Depression: Design of a Randomized Controlled Trial', *BMC Public Health*, 10, pp. 558–???.

Jamison, K. R. (1997) 'Manic-Depressive Illness and Creativity', *Scientific American*, 276, pp. 44–52.

Kant, I. (1998) *Critique of Pure Reason*, P. Guyer & A. W. Wood, eds. Cambridge, UK: Cambridge University Press.

Kharkhurin, A. V. (2014) 'Creativity. 4in1: Four-criterion Construct of Creativity', *Creativity Research Journal*, 26(3), pp. 338–352.

Klein, M. (1929) 'Infantile Anxiety-Situations Reflected in a Work of Art and in the Creative Impulse', *International Journal of Psycho-Analysis*, 10, pp. 436–443.

Kris, E. (1952) *Psychoanalytic Explorations in Art*. New York: International Universities Press.

Kristeva, J. (2005) 'L'impudence D'énoncer: La Langue Maternelle', *Revue Française de Psychanalyse*, 69, pp. 1655–1667.

Kupfer, D. J., Frank, E., & Phillips, M. L. (2012) 'Major Depressive Disorder: New Clinical, Neurobiological, and Treatment Perspectives', *The Lancet*, 379(9820), pp. 1045–1055.

Lacan, J. (1991) *The Seminar. Book II: The Ego in Freud's Theory and in the Technique of Psychoanalysis (1954–1955)*, trans. F. Last, ed. F. Last. New York: W. W. Norton & Company.

Lacan, J. (1992) *The Seminar. Book VII: The Ethics of Psychoanalysis (1959–1960)*, trans. F. LAST, ed. J.-A. Miller. New-York: W. W. Norton & Company.

Lacan, J. (1997) *The Seminar. Book III: The Psychoses (1955–1956)*, trans. F. Last, ed. J.-A. Miller. New York: W. W. Norton & Company.

Lacan, J. (1998) *The Seminar. Book XX: Encore: On Feminine Sexuality, the Limits of Love and Knowledge (1972–1973)*, trans. F. Last, ed. J.-A. Miller. New York: W. W. Norton & Company.

Lacan, J. (2001) *The Seminar. Book XI: The Four Fundamental Concepts of Psychoanalysis (1964)*, trans. F. Last, ed, J.-A. Miler. New York: W. W. Norton & Company.

Lacan, J. (2006) *Écrits*, ed, B. Fink. New York: W. W. Norton & Company.

Lacan, J. (2014) *The Seminar. Book X: Anxiety (1962–1963)*, trans. F. Last, ed. J.-A. Miller. Cambridge, UK: Polity.

Lacan, J. (2016) *The Seminar of Jacques Lacan, Book XXIII, The Sinthome (1975–1976)*, J.-A. Miller, ed. Cambridge, UK: Polity.

Lacan, J. (2017a) *The Seminar. Book V: The Formations of the Unconscious (1957–1958)*, trans. F. LAST, ed. F. Last. Cambridge, UK: Polity.

Lacan, J. (2017b) *The Seminar. Book VIII: Transference (1960–1961)*, trans. F. Last, ed, J.-A. Miler. Cambridge, UK: Polity.

Lacan, J. (2019) *The Seminar. Book VI: Desire and its Interpretation (YEAR-YEAR)*, trans. F. Last, ed. F. Last. Cambridge, UK: Polity.

Lim, G. Y., Tam, W. W., Lu, Y., Ho, C. S., Zhang, M. W., & Ho, R. C. (2018) 'Prevalence of Depression in the Community from 30 Countries between 1994 and 2014', *Scientific Reports*, 8, pp. 1–10.

Ludwig, A. M. (1992) 'The Creative Achievement Scale', *Creativity Research Journal*, 5, pp. 109–119.

Lombroso, C. (1895) *The Man of Genius*. London: W. Scott.

Miller, J. A. (2016) The Unconscious and the Speaking Body. Proceedings from: The Speaking Body, 10th Congress of the World Association of Psychoanalysis, pp. 1–11.

Opbroek, A., Delgado, P. L., Laukes, C., McGahuey, C., Katsanis, J., Moreno, F. A., & Manber, R. (2002) 'Emotional Blunting Associated with SSRI-induced Sexual Dysfunction. Do SSRIs Inhibit Emotional Responses?', *The International Journal of Neuropsychopharmacology*, 5, pp. 147–151.

Oremland, J. D. (1997) *The Origins and Psychodynamics of Creativity: A Psychoanalytic Perspective*. Madison: International Universities Press, Inc.

Post, F. (1996) 'Verbal Creativity, Depression and Alcoholism. An Investigation of One Hundred American and British Writers', *The British Journal of Psychiatry*, 168, pp. 545–555.

Prentky, R. A. (2001) 'Mental Illness and Roots of Genius', *Creativity Research Journal*, 13, pp. 95–104.

Price, J., & Goodwin, G. M. (2009) 'Emotional Blunting or Reduced Reactivity Following Remission of Major Depression', *Medicographia*, 31, pp. 152–156.

Reynolds, M. W., Nabors, L., & Quinlan, A. (2000) 'The Effectiveness of Art Therapy: Does it Work?', *Art Therapy*, 17, pp. 207–213.

Roudinesco, E. (1997) *Jacques Lacan*. New York: Columbia University Press.

Roussillon, R. (2005) 'Le Processus et la Capacité Sublimatoire', *Revue Française de Psychanalyse*, 69, pp. 1565–1573.

Runco, M. A., & Jaeger, G. J. (2012) 'The Standard Definition of Creativity', *Creativity Research Journal*, 24, pp. 92–96.

Salguero, J. M., Extremera, N., & Fernández-Berrocal, P. (2012) 'Emotional Intelligence and Depression: The Moderator Role of Gender', *Personality and Individual Differences*, 53, pp. 29–32.

Silvia, P. J., & Kimbrel, N. A. (2010) 'A Dimensional Analysis of Creativity and Mental Illness: Do Anxiety and Depression Symptoms Predict Creative Cognition, Creative Accomplishments, and Creative Self-concepts?', *Psychology of Aesthetics, Creativity, and the Arts*, 4, pp. 2–10.

Stavrakakis, Y. (2007) 'Antinomies of Creativity: Lacan and Castoriadis on Social Construction and the Political', *The Lacanian Left: Essays on Psychoanalysis and Politics*, 37, pp. 37–65.

Vanheule, S. (2011) *The Subject of Psychosis: A Lacanian Perspective*. New York: Springer.

Weisberg, R. W. (2015) 'On the Usefulness of 'Value' in the Definition of Creativity', *Creativity Research Journal*, 27, pp. 111–124.

Žižek, S. (2000) 'Melancholy and the Act', *Critical Inquiry*, 26(4), 657–681.

Chapter 10

Dressing up the death drive

Mourning as a defense against melancholia

Jamieson Webster and Patricia Gherovici

The recent work on terrorism by the French psychoanalyst Genevieve Morel (2018) on people who turned themselves in to the French authorities instead of committing suicide bombings offers insights that allow us to make helpful clinical distinctions about melancholy in psychosis and hysteria. In her various examples, Morel highlights the contrasts between the act of suicide-murder and the ideals fueling them. Melancholia is a crucial aspect in these cases, as these planned acts concerned an inevitable failure of sublimation. Facing a depressive warding off of anxiety, the necessary psychical work of mourning was circumvented through the planned acts of violence. In some of the cases she explores, the move from plan to action was effectively avoided by engaging in creative works such as writing, participating in politics, finding religion, or beginning love affairs.

Morel (2018) reminds us of many writers who, when the writing stopped, committed suicide – a recent example being David Foster Wallace. If we follow her hypothesis, writing seems to function merely as a momentary deferral of a move into action or a *passage à l'acte*. The only time when this does not happen, according to Morel, is when toxicomania is part of the clinical picture – that is, when the person's melancholia is intertwined with addiction. If they become sober, they can continue to live, irrespective of engaging in creative or other work of redemption. Getting rid of the addiction is a life-saver. This observation was quite surprising and left open a number of questions. Where does mourning fit into this picture of melancholia in tension with creativity? Is creativity, as it has often been observed, a form of mourning? With melancholic authors, is the work of writing simply a defense against mourning, a deferral of melancholia, and not necessarily a proper work of mourning, as the grieving of a loss, as it might be for others?

Let us take a little detour. Elaine Scarry, who famously wrote *The Body in Pain: The Making and Unmaking of the World* (1987), has also written a fascinating book on creativity – *Dreaming by The Book* (2001). Her main claim is that if you look closely at literature and poetry, the text is not only about the imagination of an author put into language, but a sort of instruction manual that transmits to the reader the task and properties of imagination itself. Every description is not merely the description – at times beautiful, painful, or wonderous – of a scene,

DOI: 10.4324/9781003216391-11

object, or person (or combination thereof), but in fact what it takes psychically to perceive these in one's mind, to verbally give the scene something that approximates reality or real perception. For example, in Thomas Hardy's *Tess of the D'Ubervilles* the reader, she says, is instructed through a typical pastoral image – cows in a dairy – in the art of imagination:

> The sun, lowering itself, behind this patient row, threw their shadows accurately inwards upon the wall. Thus it threw shadows of these obscure and homely figures every evening with as much care over each contour as if it had been the profile of a court beauty on a palace wall; copied them as diligently as it had copied Olympian shapes on marble facades long ago, or the outline of Alexander, Caesar, and the Pharaohs.
>
> (Scarry, 2001, p. 19)

Scarry points out that regardless of whether we want to commit to Hardy's metaphor of the shadows of cows upon the dairy wall channeling Greek, Roman, and Egyptian civilization, what is evoked is the act of making – making a metaphor that is also the metaphor itself. The labor of constructing is here named "care."

What is marked out is the relation between figure and ground, screen and projection, object and light, solidity and ephemerality, as well as, the extension of body and mind in time (the time of light, of the sun lowering, but also every evening) and space (patient row, palace wall, marble facades). The image or scene also moves: "sun, lowering itself," "threw their shadows accurately inwards," "care over each contour," and "copied them as diligently." Yet, this action is something that seems to happen, without the intervention of our will, in the subjunctive tense, or middle voice. The hand or eyes want to catch up with the scene, which is a scene of the mimesis of aliveness. What is important is the life of an object: the life experienced in relation to an object that becomes the capacity for imagination.

For Scarry, this is about interiorization – "a yearning to incorporate, to make a residual image" and the "formal properties of this act are displayed in the content of its object" (Scarry, 2001, p. 66). This is not, importantly, a putting of mind onto the object, but the reverse, the object put to the mind. The nimbleness with which we can set an object in motion depends on having this materiality: can we fold it, tilt it, make it radiant, make it circle, whirl, tilt, skate? Can we invest in it, or allow this investment to come forth? This is also for Scarry a constant act of composition and recomposition: hence the affinity with the arts and not simply "reality." This is how she defines the sense of vivacity that is transmitted through art, through this secret instruction manual on creativity. In this way, it is a contribution to the social fabric.

Take the following example from Homer's *Iliad*. It shows not only the flash of light against bronze, the fire used to craft armor and weapon, and the passion that ignites humans, especially in love and war, but also speaks to the spark of imagination present in work, the way the mind and body wheels around themselves, reeling as a central axis and its pivot, much as the image of men rushing forth across the earth.

> Glistening burnished helmets shone, streaming out of the ships … The glory of armor lit the skies and the whole earth laughed, rippling under the glitter of bronze … And in their midst the brilliant Achilles began to arm for battle …
>   Three times the brilliant Achilles gave his war cry over the trench, three times the Trojans and famous allies whirled in panic—
>   Helmet flashing, Hector wheeled with a dark glance.
>
> (Homer, 1998, p.19)

Yes, ostensibly *Iliad* is a description of war and battle, but it is also about mourning and loss, about memorializing, and reckoning with human violence and destruction. It is also a long depiction of the care with which we treat corpses. This can be seen when the body of Hector is anointed and placed on the mourning wagon:

> And white-armed Andromache led their songs of sorrow, cradling the head of Hector, man-killing Hector gently in her arms … all his brothers, his friends-in-arms, mourning, and warm tears come streaming down their cheeks. They placed the bones they found in a golden chest, shrouding them round and round in soft purple cloth.
>
> (Homer, 1998, p. 24)

While it is the care with which we treat a corpse, this action also speaks to creativity and mourning. The men whirl, and Hector wheels. The wheels of the mourning wagon turn and turn, the body is cradled, shrouded, round and round, tears are streaming: this is both a scene and song of mourning, the turning of the object over and over in one's mind, even the violence and pain with which it lodges itself there, with which we rush at it, and also the swift movement with which it can leave us.

We would not be far from Freud's famous statement in *Mourning and Melancholia* (1919) that, during mourning, the object is reconstituted before it is given up, that every trace, every libidinal attachment, every interiorized connection to the object must be re-traversed, in order to give the judgment, alive as this representation in my mind, this meaning that the object holds for me, but now dead in reality, a corpse, gone. This composition must take place over time to accept the loss of the object by a mind which does not know death. Only then can a life with a new object take place.

We are pretty squarely here in the territory of creativity on the side of the work of mourning, *Eros*, life, rending, and mending of the social fabric. We are even speaking about the transmission of the capacity for vivacity, however much it relies on the acceptance of the loss or lack of the object and assuming some part of the responsibility for its destruction. But what about melancholia? A patient once dreamt that a slide that she was on was a waterslide: its end was closed and so was filled up with water, which meant that by the time she reached the bottom, she would drown. She realized the joke in the dream, or rather the pun – *suislide*. The dream is a dream where nothing holds, everything metonymically slides. The death drive in full stride.

In another dream of a patient, she saw her mother's severed arm, inert, almost mannequin-like, even more dead and unreal than a violently torn object. Behind this, was the image she had seen that day of an actor who, surprisingly, kissed the arm of his co-actress on the red carpet in front of a large bank of paparazzi cameras. This became an internet sensation. The image, the kiss, the sign of desire, the sensation even, was certainly not interiorized as alive in this dream. The atmosphere in the dream renders the object dead, Eros suddenly turning to its opposite.

Something of this melancholic scene of mortification can be found in Sylvia Plath's *Poem for a Birthday – The Stones,* which stands in stark contrast to the imagery used by Elaine Scarry. Plath is of course a notorious melancholic who ended her life by suicide. The poem begins:

> This is the city where men are mended.
> I lie on a great anvil.
> The flat blue sky-circle
>
> Flew off like the hat of a doll
> When I fell out of the light. I entered
> The stomach of indifference, the wordless cupboard.
>
> The mother of pestles diminished me.
> I became a still pebble.
> The stones of the belly were peaceable,
>
> The head-stone quiet, jostled by nothing.
> Only the mouth-hole piped out,
> Importunate cricket.

(Plath, 2008, p. 136)

The spark, the sudden ignition of light, the beginning manipulation of space and objects, happens in reverse: the sky is flat and flies off, she falls out of the light, enters indifference, wordlessness, and is diminished. She is the object – she does not have an object. Everything is still and doesn't move – the beautiful contradiction of being "jostled by nothing." The mouth is a hole that pipes out sounds like a cricket – not a war cry that makes one whirl, not a song of sorrow, nor a scene of mourning, but sliding into the abyss.

The poem continues as all of this leads to what Plath calls an after-hell, a city of spare parts, of which she is but one amongst them. More and more we are in the realm of dead objects,

This is the after-hell: I see the light.
A wind unstoppers the chamber
Of the ear, old worrier.

Water mollifies the flint lip,
And daylight lays its sameness on the wall.
The grafters are cheerful,

Heating the pincers, hoisting the delicate hammers.
A current agitates the wires
Volt upon volt. Catgut stitches my fissures.

A workman walks by carrying a pink torso.
The storerooms are full of hearts.
This is the city of spare parts.

(Plath, 2008, p. 137)

The failure of the imagination is ever-present – "the current agitates the wire." It is an instruction manual on the inability to give vivacity to objects: "The daylight lays its sameness on the wall." This is a city of severed arms, of hearts as spare parts in a stockroom. Love is dead material, "bone," "bald," "sinew," "curse."

You can reconstruct, compose, re-compose, mend, and stitch, but these are just the covering for an emptiness. In fact, she says that space is an empty house for an elusive rose, a bowl for nothing but shadows. There is nothing to do. This isn't *even* hell – that was the diminishment upon the anvil as the world flew off. This is an after-hell, of greeting the world, "I see the light", to find no real object. This is the birthday in the birthday poem. Time in this crypt does not lead to reparation; or the reparation on offer – the food tubes, the spare parts – is worse than being "jostled by nothing."

The difference between literature that speaks to the imagination and therefore also time and space, and at times, mourning, and melancholic work, seems as clear as the day. One is an attempt at interiorizing the object, while this poem of pure melancholia is the refusal of mourning and the feeling of being the object and not having or interiorizing any object. And yet, how can we say that this isn't creative, that it isn't staggeringly beautiful? Of course, we cannot. What would it mean then as psychoanalysts to diagnose the poem melancholic, however easy it would be to do so given the tragic fate of Sylvia Plath? In the context of psychoanalysis, would we not be seeking somehow to cure this melancholia? To find another birthday?

Sylvia Plath, in the poem, is stitched, mended, and given objects, but these are false cures and dead objects. They may even be repetitive, violent, traumatic objects. She sees them as a kind of ruse–perhaps engineered by capitalism and patriarchy. The death drive in Plath feels palpable, it speaks to violence inside of life that is intertwined with loss and makes difficult the possibility of living. This, for example, doesn't seem to be true of the world of Homer or Hardy, however violent those worlds may be at times. For Plath then, life, objects, are represented as brute materiality that one cannot move, words calling out in a vacuum, or its opposite, the world as flying off, the subject as falling endlessly, the mind as painfully unstoppered. Neither of these is a motion that one can move with, be moved by, and the poem is like the subject hanging on, by the slightest hook or thread.

Even if psychoanalysis tries to offer a possibility: the possibility of living, of moving, of speaking, we must wrestle always with the death drive and its appearance in life, to know where to begin to try and protect a patient, and to offer 'care'. Psychoanalysis can be the place of a real encounter, something we can turn round and round in our minds, that ignites the spark of desire. Let us say this: its possibility is there in Plath, however negated it is. She is, in this poem, searching for it, perhaps best found in the solidity of the anvil, the still pebble, the peaceable stone, indeed the cupboard, all which appear before the after-hell, the world of simulacra. Even the dissatisfaction with those objects points to a satisfaction yearned for, maybe even somewhere known or remembered.

The problem, or at least the importance of psychoanalysis, is that someone has to hear it, to begin to gently lay their hands around a patient *there*, and help them to move ever so slightly. It will change her writing, and there would be great resistance to that – many analysts have faced these crossroads in analytic work. And in the end, the difficulty is that the choice between life and death is more the patient's than it would be the psychoanalyst's. We can only continue to lend our ears, to fight to hear, as long as they continue to come and speak to us.

A testimony of this transformation is given by a recent memoir by philosopher and psychoanalytic theorist, Richard Boothby (2022), titled *Blown Away: Refinding Life After My Son's Suicide*. Boothby describes the moment that he emerges from two years of painful mourning, a year, as he put it, of shock, endless crying, and pure pain, and then a second year, somehow numb and wrecked, in an even worse state. Pursuing the guilt with which he lacerated himself, session after session, he finally acknowledged his disavowed violence, something he came to from a forgotten memory from childhood of participating in the act of killing a helpless turtle. This somehow allowed him to emerge from the endless state of numb pain. The truth about himself that he had misrecognized didn't necessarily explain his son's suicide, something he desperately wanted the analysis to do, but it did mean acknowledging that they shared a violence. He felt closer to his son.

With the death drive brought to the surface, his memories of his son suddenly took on an aliveness, as if he was there conversing with him, feeling even the physical weight of his body when they hugged. This didn't lessen the pain, in fact, it intensified it, showing him what was gone. But it was also a new son, or a new sense of his son, more alive for what he didn't understand about him, just as he hadn't understood himself. It was as if the liveliness of the memories was being fueled by the discovery of this lack, bringing him closer to his son than they had ever been. It is this process that he wanted to write in the form of a book.

What we can see in this example is that analysis gives room to the death drive that was fueling the melancholia, and marks it through traversal of memories and fantasies that, as Boothby says, did not correspond to his sense of himself, his ego. It takes his ego apart, and with it, the object (in this case his son) that is then put together anew. In fact, the work with the death drive marks their radical separation from one another, in life and in death. But this mystery begins to be a source of life, vivacity, and one might even say desire. It is also a moment of internalizing his son in a new way. At the very least, the desire becomes a desire to write this book, honor his son, and, as he said, continue living and not follow him into death.

Is sublimation, tied to mourning and the internalization of the object, a defense against melancholia? Is it a dressing-up of the death drive? Is most creative work on the brink of melancholia, a sometimes more, sometimes less, successful deferral of it? Let us turn to another, more bleak, example of melancholia in a parent-child couple, and its creative expression. Fashion designer Alexander McQueen's Metropolitan Museum of Art show, *Savage Beauty*, was one of the ten most popular shows in the museum's history and attracted 650,000 visitors, 15,000 alone on the day before it closed.

When the final days of the already-extended show approached, crowds gathered, waiting for hours in the rain, in a line that emulated a fashion runway, visitors dressed in outfits that quoted McQueen's signature style. The exhibition's amazing success cannot be explained by the media frenzy around the wedding gown worn by a future queen, Kate Middleton, from McQueen's studio, the story of his truncated life, nor even the contagious nature of fashion fads. In fact, it seems as if something about its designer's melancholia is what fascinated the audience.

In fact, the exhibition was quite overwhelming. We might characterize the show as one that moves between the adjective "savage" and the verb "ravage." One goes to 'Savage Beauty' knowing that McQueen killed himself the night before his mother's funeral, that he was found dead in his wardrobe, that he took a huge overdose of drugs, slashed his wrists with a ceremonial dagger and a meat cleaver, and hanged himself. It was well known that he suffered from depression. The show seduced by offering itself as a lasting riddle.

McQueen, unable to cope with the loss of his beloved mother, Joyce, committed suicide on the eve of her burial. The family considered postponing her funeral and burying mother and son together. After agonizing deliberations, this did not happen, mainly because of a delay caused by the police inquest on the cause of his death, which was eventually confirmed as suicide. In life, McQueen and his mother had been extremely close. They appeared together in a Guardian interview in 2004 in which the mother asked her son: "What is your most terrifying fear?" to which he replied, "Dying before you." His mother quipped, "Thank you, son." She asked, "What makes you proud?" He responded, "You."

When McQueen announced the news of his mother's demise on his Twitter feed, the phrase read like his own death sentence: "I'm letting my followers know my mother passed away yesterday if it she had not me nor would you RIP mumxxxxxxxxxxxxxxxxxxxxxxxxxxxxxxx ..." McQueen seemed to exhort his fans to honor and be grateful to the woman who had given birth to him, but the sentence can also mean that she still had this son, as if a separation between mother and child had not yet taken place. Unable to extricate himself from his mother, the fusion exacted its toll. If she no longer had him, no one would.

After his suicide, one may read the message's repeated letter "x," written with no space after the word "mum," as a failed attempt at delineating what Lacan calls *objet petit a*, the object-cause of desire, the unfathomable X on account of which we desire. The status of this enigmatic object, alive, unknowable, may be the key to understanding why some people manage to mourn their loss and find a substitute whereas others remain inconsolable and refuse to let go of the lost object – in some cases, following it to death.

The lost object is not the same in mourning and in melancholia: "Mourning is regularly the reaction to the loss of a loved person, or to the loss of some abstraction which has taken the place of one, such as one's country, liberty, an ideal, and so on" (Freud, 1917, p. 234). Whereas in melancholy,

> the object has not perhaps actually died but has been lost as an object of love ... . In yet other cases one feels justified in maintaining the belief that a loss of this kind has occurred, but one cannot see clearly what it is that has been lost ... . This would suggest that melancholia is in some way related to an object-loss which is withdrawn from consciousness, in contradiction to mourning, in which there is nothing about the loss that is unconscious.
>
> (Freud, 1917, p. 245)

For the mourner, it is the lack of the object that causes the suffering, whereas, for the melancholic subject, the object of grievance is not really lost but rather maintained within the subject, buried alive in the ego, from where it remains and causes intense suffering, becoming a devouring vortex of pain.

Freud sums this up with his usual eloquence: "In mourning it is the world that has become empty; in melancholia it is the ego itself" (Freud, 1917, p. 246). For Freud, because melancholics cannot encounter what they have lost in the object, that is, what in the object caused their desire, they cannot begin the "bit-by-bit" psychical symbolic work of mourning. The melancholic identifies with and holds onto the lost, abandoned, or dead object in what Freud calls a "hallucinatory wishful psychosis."

McQueen's tragic end shares resemblances with the death of another grief-stricken son who could not continue living after losing his 84-year-old adored mother. Roland Barthes, the famous French literary critic, was devoted to his mother and lived with her all his life. The day after his mother died, he started keeping a diary of his suffering. He wrote:

> The desires I had before her death (while she was sick) can no longer be fulfilled, for that would mean it is her death that allows me to fulfill them – her

death might be a liberation in some sense with regard to my desires. But her death has changed me, I no longer desire what I used to desire. I must await – supposing that such a thing could happen – for a new desire to form, a desire following her death.

(Barthes, 2010, p. 18)

Barthes describes her loss not as the loss of a loved object but as the loss of desire itself. Unable to mourn his mother, he cannot allow a new desire to follow in the place that she has evacuated.

Eerily, in his second to last entry in his mourning journal, he writes, "Nap. Dream: exactly her smile. Dream: complete, successful, memory" (Barthes, 2010, p. 242). In the place where one might imagine that he would encounter her absence, he hallucinates, exactly, her smile. Complete. Roland Barthes died an absurd death at age 64. After leaving lunch with Francois Mitterand, France's future president, Barthes walked back home without paying attention to the traffic. He was struck by a laundry van and died, less of the injuries, which altogether were not life-threatening, than from a general depression.

The destiny of the "lost object" remains crucial here. Whether it is accepted as "lost," as in the painful process of unbinding love ties that takes place in mourning, or it is reclaimed as a gangrenous part of the ego by way of narcissistic identification, as in melancholy, one needs to keep in mind that the place of the "lost object" in fact serves as a protective screen over the abyss of the unnamable, of something impossible to imagine or comprehend; namely, what Lacan calls the Real. All lost objects (like the mother's breast or smile) are already substitutions with respect to this empty place. In light of this, one can make sense of Lacan's claim that, unbeknown to us, the "lost object" is the support of our castration and, thus, it represents what allows desire to continue. The possibility of replacing the object renders life possible. Mourning is a defense against melancholia.

Freud tells us that, for the melancholic, this loss remains unintelligible. What can be seen, he says, is the ego "overwhelmed by the object," crushed by it, much like when we are in a state of love. It is as if the object's impossible absence had caused it to grow too large. The melancholic is, therefore, not only a frustrated subject unable to detach from the lost object, longing for its return, but also a subject who, in the presence of the object itself, will always be disappointed with it. Lacan declared depression to be a kind of moral cowardice, a sentimental sadness always too much in the grip of the death drive. Lacan was worried about the nostalgia and moral masochism inherent in melancholia. In melancholia, there is a refusal not just of mourning but of desire, and with it, a refusal of the lack that perpetuates it. Lacan explains mourning not simply in terms of identification with the lost object but in relation to lack. "We mourn but for he of whom we can say *I was his lack* [*j'etais son manque*]. We mourn people that we have treated either well or badly, but with respect to whom we don't know that we fulfilled the function of being in the place of their lack" (Lacan, 2014, p. 141). Lacan alerts us that mourning concerns having been or not an object for the Other at the place of their lack.

For that object (*objet a*, object-cause of desire) to exist, a separation needs to have occurred, a cut necessary for life to be possible, carving out a space between oneself and one's own sadness, between oneself and this other to whom melancholics offer themselves up as an object, which is, from one angle, the work of psychoanalysis. Nevertheless, it is precisely because of the near hallucinatory concatenation, that the cut posited by Lacan as central to the psychoanalytic act is so incredibly difficult with the melancholic. Self-laceration, the abnegation of the melancholic, is one attempt to introduce a cut, to encounter the scene of one's desire, and one that often fails, or succeeds – to turn it around – only at its limits in the act of suicide.

Returning to McQueen, Freud and Lacan's theories of melancholia help to explain the experience of attending his show. The overall effect of his work is mesmerizing. He has "the" object and shows it to us, magnified and dressed in its gaudy guises. The beauty, and perhaps the attraction, is to render the experience of this melancholic tie in this sublime fashion, to bury you beneath it. Through his work, we tolerate (barely, at times; our breath seems to leave us midway) this deadly, sinister, claustrophobic space after which is only life, loss, and the comings and goings of desire. In McQueen's theatrical runway shows, the model's body is delivered to us as a site of persecution, indeed of an experience at this limit, a kind of painful pleasure (*jouissance*), which can be viewed by us precisely because of the magnificence of the clothing or the setting that veils it – this is what is savage about beauty.

After having toured McQueen's show, it was not surprising that he committed suicide by hanging himself. Too many of the images play with being irrevocably tied, the presence of a deadly umbilicus to an object whose image is always on the border of life and death, and the inability to breathe. There is his Kate Moss angel hologram, more ominous than joyful. Or the wallpaper where babies appear in a state of fragmentation, tied to figures with gas masks and to images of poisonous nature. Think of the infamous reenactment of Joel-Peter Witkin's photograph, "Sanitarium" – a woman breathing through a tube in a box filled with moths in McQueen's last show.

Aside from all of the beauty of this exhibition, savage or otherwise, what also lingered was something of this "false morality" in melancholia that Lacan highlights, best seen in his oscillation between helpless romanticism, techno progressivism, and a glorified nihilism – all exacting a kind of external domination. McQueen doesn't trust the desire of his viewer, nor does he trust desire itself. Thus, his show is not so much about the creation of an opening in desire, but rather a means of turning back to the audience the death drive that has swept desire away.

The tirade against fashion, which he displayed on his runway as a full garbage heap, models dragging around remnants like carcasses, his stark plaid collections that rage against his mother country, as well as the endlessly victimized women verging on the comic, are perhaps a few of the more successful examples of his works of "false morality." But, from our perspective, much of it was too glib.

More room for desire might have allowed his audience more of a place in relation to his work.

McQueen's fashion, in its refined ingenuity, shows an evolution toward a more successful and encompassing sublimation by freeing itself more and more from what seemed gratuitous in the first attempts which we see as linked to the death drive. It was this, McQueen the master tailor and textural genius, the recycler of worn-out images high and low, the re-inventor of the boundaries between fashion and theater, and his relentless pursuit of imaging the limits of pleasure and of bodily form, that one wanted to wrest from the grip and fixity of the death drive. You feel as if you can imagine its possibility had he lived; you feel, in the crevices of the crowds and in spite of their overblown performance of rapture, the more delicate sublimity of his work. It would be a fashion that would read more like a text, more of an appeal than a statement.

Lacan always felt that when speech was reduced to a statement or sign, we were doomed to the sadistic voyeuristic complex at the heart of one's ego, something that plays its fair share in the cruelty of depression. Desire, signification, and, indeed, sublimation as tied to mourning and the life of the object, has to be something else, somewhere else. But many seem to be looking in McQueen, not for sublimation, but for the sublime as a way to experience this foreclosed, savage, melancholic space, dressed and rendered beautifully. McQueen, in the end, refused to give up the object and, being unable to give up the crown, refusing to abdicate, died on the throne of his own creation.

Thinking of the title of this exhibition, the word "savage" brought to mind Samuel Beckett's reflections on his mother: "I am what her savage loving made me, and it is good that one of us should accept that finally" (Bair, 1990, p. 263). One could add to this the title of one of his most beautiful short stories, "Enough," a story about love that grows old and drags; a love whose beauty, in a state of waning, is, finally, enough. One cannot help but link this possibility to him having had enough of her, and, perhaps, to having had psychoanalysis with Bion, the conclusion of which was to finally leave "Ireland" behind. With it, a crippling depression also left.

If Beckett's work is savage at times, it is also deeply funny and optimistic, without a trace of moralism or sentimentality. Perhaps this is, sadly, the inverse tale to that of Alexander McQueen, the possibility that comes with having cut the rope. Beckett's is a love of beauty in decline, not in an overwhelming, hypertrophied, crushing excess. Perhaps this is one way of defining the line between art and mere fashions. As Cocteau said, "Art produces ugly things which frequently become more beautiful with time. Fashion, on the other hand, produces beautiful things which always become ugly with time." One wishes that the beauty of the show would not have been so captious that it veiled the sadness that would lead to mourning. One wishes McQueen could have said "Enough!" in a less lethal manner. Paradoxically, however, the relationship to fashion is always predicated on the not-enough. How else could we explain the exclamation, "I have nothing to wear!" while facing an overflowing closet?

In conclusion, if melancholia is seeking a limit, to break from the object that it keeps by maintaining it lodged in the ego, the creation of this boundary is not always encountered through acts of sublimation. Sublimation rather reflects the unique limits of the way by which existence is possible. Sublimation, as we saw with McQueen, is a way of dressing up the will to create from zero, the "nothing" of the death drive. But this escape valve for *jouissance* collapses when McQueen's mother actually dies. Identified with her, he loses himself as well. To lose and survive the loss, a new position must be claimed on the side of mourning, tolerating the death that sustains and frames with the veil of fantasy the vivacity of objects, allowing us to enjoy the play of the unconscious, not simply, or only, showing us the enjoyment of the symptom, which, in the case of melancholia, can be quite deadly.

We know that psychoanalytically, wresting the subject from the grip of the death drive is difficult. There is no guarantee that this will even be possible. One can see melancholic productions as trying to construct a space, to break open the fixity of the death drive (even as too much slippage). One should listen psychoanalytically, as it were, for the place of desire, for the cut. But that is only one way of hearing melancholic creations because the enjoyment of a work's foreclosure is always also possible, the audience or reader of the work contagiously feeling the pulse of the death drive. This is where, for both artist and audience, the work only contributes to the foreclosure of mourning.

The gamble of psychoanalysis resides in helping the analysand to move from a melancholic position by creating a hole, an interval, a space, to break away from the death drive's grip and allow the object *a* to be extracted. This is hard work, not just for the analyst, but most importantly for the analysand. If this happens, there will be room for an invention, for a stable creation that will not just fuel the melancholia. Here Lacan's notion of sinthome is helpful. The work of analysis implies not just a yielding of *jouissance*; it is not simply about the fall of an illusion or traversal of a fundamental fantasy but rather the constitution of something new, a sinthome, that is, the creation of a new symptom that does not need to be cured.

In melancholy, the necrotized object threatens to infect the whole subject ultimately making life unsustainable; the work of analysis is aimed at moving away from the deadly excess of *jouissance* that makes the object all too real. For McQueen, there was nothing to stop the confusion between the loss of his mother and the loss of lack that makes desire and life possible. Without engaging with psychobiography, this may call up Plath about to turn the gas on and put her head in the oven to kill herself in the early morning, having sealed the kitchen door with tape and towels as if to protect her children sleeping in the next room. Nevertheless, she was putting them in peril – an explosion could have happened. Her children nearby, not yet her object *a* as a prime mover of desire, were at risk of being dragged down from the scene altogether in her suicidal *passage à l'acte*.

It is not the art of dying, succumbing to the siren call of the death drive, as in Plath's poem "Lady Lazarus," but rather developing the art of living with the death drive. Not only has psychoanalysis a hystericizing effect but the direction of the cure aims at a necessary traversal of mourning, as proposed by Serge Leclaire in *A Child Is Being Killed* (1998), which means getting rid of the narcissistically invested fantastic mirage of ourselves that has been implanted in us by our parents. Only once the work of mourning is achieved, once the salutary loss that will permit someone to enjoy their sinthome is accepted, then life becomes livable.

References

Bair, D. (1990) *Samuel Beckett: A Biography*. New York: Simon and Schuster.

Barthes, R. (2010) *Mourning Diary*, trans. R. Howard. New York: Hill and Wang.

Boothby, R. (2022) *Blown Away: Refinding Life After My Son's Suicide*. New York: Other Press.

Freud, S. (1917) 'Mourning and Melancholia', In J. Strachey (Ed.), *The Standard Edition of the Complete Psychological Works of Sigmund Freud*, Volume 14. London: The Hogarth Press and the Institute of Psycho-Analysis. 239–260.

Homer. (1998) *The Iliad*, trans. R. Fagles. New York: Penguin.

Lacan, J. (2014). *The Seminar Book X: Anxiety* (translated by A.R. Price). J.-A. Miller (Ed.). Cambridge: Polity.

Leclaire, S. (1998) *A Child is Being Killed: On Primary Narcissism and the Death Drive*. Stanford: Stanford University Press.

Morel, G. (2018) *Terroristes: Les Raisons Intimes d'un Fléau Global*. Paris: Fayard.

Plath, S. (2008) *The Collected Poems*. New York: Harper Collins.

Scarry, E. (1987) *The Body in Pain: The Making and Unmaking of the World*. Oxford: Oxford University Press.

Scarry, E (2001) *Dreaming by the Book*. Princeton: Princeton University Press.

Chapter 11

The specificity of manic-depressive psychosis

Darian Leader

Clinicians working in a Lacanian framework will be familiar with three main diagnostic categories of psychosis: paranoia, melancholia and schizophrenia. All predicated on the mechanism of foreclosure, they tend to be differentiated in terms of the relation to the Other, the treatment of morbid excitation and the establishment of meaning. Depressive states outside melancholia are considered on a case-by-case basis, and the same can largely be said for periods of elation and exuberance.

But what of manic-depressive psychosis? One of the central categories of classical psychiatry, Lacan had nonetheless little to say about it as a nosological entity, whether through acknowledgement or critique. There are a few references in the early psychiatric work, and later some comments on mania and depression in his seminars and writings. These are often quoted, yet the actual question of the diagnostic category has received far less attention. Despite the fact that the label of manic-depressive psychosis is used in clinical presentations, there seem to be no real distinguishing features beyond the standard conceptualisations of foreclosure and mania.

And this brings us to our first problem: even the most cursory reading of Lacan's remarks on these themes gives a clinical picture which is, to say the least, non-specific. The comments on mania, for example, apply just as much to the states of intense agitation and verbal association found in schizophrenia as they do to the so-called 'flight of ideas' of manic-depression. The remarks on 'manic excitation', on the other hand, could qualify just as well certain forms of hallucination or perturbations within the field of affects. And when Lacan uses the term adjectively to qualify the experience of the end of the analysis, he is clearly not suggesting a diagnostic judgement.

A similar difficulty is found in Freud's work. In 'Mourning and Melancholia' he includes mania with melancholia, despite the fact that clinically the occurrence of melancholias that never generate manias is far more frequent. Indeed, there are many reasons to question Freud's polarisation, and the cautious tone of his text seems justified. It could be argued that the lows of manic-depression are fundamentally different from those of melancholia, with far less fixity on a single motif, and, equally, that the phenomenology of manic-depression is much closer to schizophrenia than it is to melancholia.

DOI: 10.4324/9781003216391-12

As we start thinking about these questions, a number of clinical and conceptual problems are raised which might help us to consider more critically our use of diagnostic categories and the delimitations we make between them. First, let's look at some historical issues.

*

Just as analysts tend to claim a special atemporal pedigree for hysteria, so psychiatrists frequently accord a comparable place to manic-depression. Citations from Aretaeus of Cappadocia inevitably precede excerpts from medieval writers on accidie, and a line is sketched from the classical world to Kraepelin's clinic of late nineteenth century Germany and then on to the bipolar disorders of today. The clinical phenomena of exaltation and dejection are taken to indicate a historical unity as if all documented descriptions were circumscribing the same form of human distress.

Yet these ubiquitous histories are rather misleading. Note, first of all, that the endlessly iterated Aretaeus quotations always contain points of ellipsis which, if filled in, present both a varying clinical picture and confirmation that the Greek writer was not trying to frame a distinct diagnostic category. Medieval notions of accidie are similarly decontextualised and linked far too casually to contemporary theories of depression. Indeed, medieval writers frequently associate accidie with gossiping and diversion rather than the stupor and silence we might hope for. But the key discontinuity here is really to be found in pre-Kraepelinian psychiatry and especially in the work of Jean-Pierre Falret (1854) and Jules Baillarger (1854).

It was well-recognised in mid-nineteenth-century psychiatry that states of acute depression and elation could be found in any number of diagnostic structures. From the 1840s onwards, there was an effort to distinguish a specific clinical entity that involved a sequential passage through such states from the many other clinical forms that alienists had documented. Falret's circular madness and Baillarger's double-form madness were formulations of this entity, although both authors admitted that they had only ever seen a handful of cases.

In contrast to the mainstream psychiatry of today, they were trying to move beyond the question of mood fluctuations to study the quality of such states, the relation between them and the thought processes underlying them. In agreement with many of their contemporaries, they argued that mania and melancholia were in no way diagnostic of the entity they were describing. A manic episode or a melancholic depression would not point to a diagnosis of circular or double-form madness, and the new categories were introduced precisely to make this point.

With Kraepelin, this careful work would be sadly undone. Starting from the sixth edition of his 'Psychiatry', he forged a notion of 'manic-depressive insanity' which annexed nearly all manias and melancholias to manic-depression, regardless of rhythm or sequence, as well as all forms of periodic and circular psychosis. Despite hundreds of critiques, many given impetus by the hostility to German scholarship after the first war, this reductionist view eventually achieved a certain dominance in American psychiatry. The bipolar diagnoses of today often cite

Kraepelin as their historical precedent and certainly share with him an enthusiasm for over-inclusiveness. But we should note that, contrary to the usual claims, Kraepelin had no concept of affective disorders, and he makes hardly any reference at all to problems of mood.

Now, if Kraepelin at first had divided the psychoses into two main groups – manic-depression and dementia praecox – by 1920, he was not so sure (Kraepelin, 1920). Both his critics and his students had been struck by the difficulty of maintaining the differentiation. What of the manic-depressive who showed the 'symptoms' of dementia praecox – the stereotypies, the hallucinations, the negativism, the suggestibility? And what of the praecox patient who was angry and excitable at one moment, yet withdrawn and silent at the next? Interestingly, these observations tended to move from manic-depression to dementia praecox rather than the other way round, a fact echoed in the studies of diagnostic practice in the 1940s which found that a very high percentage of those diagnosed initially with manic-depression were later diagnosed with schizophrenia, although the reverse was not the case (Hoch & Rachlin, 1941).

The difficulty in differentiating certain cases of excitement as circular or schizophrenic here led to several compromise suggestions, like that of Bleuler's 'schizoid manic reactions'. Psychiatrists like Bleuler (1922), Gaupp (1925) and Courbon (1913) were interested in the intersection between the two categories, and the new label of 'combined psychosis' gained increasing currency. There was clearly a problem here. The categories were attractive, yet clinically no hard and fast distinctions could be relied on. Hence the creation of the new hybrids.

In the psychoanalytic literature, opinion was also divided. Ernest Jones was one of the first to publish a psychoanalytic study of a case of hypomania in 1909, yet a few years later would write to Freud that he doubted manic-depression really existed. In a letter of February, 1914, he admits that

> It looks to me as if there were no such disease [as manic-depressive insanity], some cases being psychoneuroses, others paraphrenia (especially paranoia), the prominence of the affective symptoms replacing the other mechanisms of distortion (as they do in dreams sometimes).
>
> (Jones, 1911, pp. 203–218)

Abraham and Klein of course wrote a great deal on this subject, yet, curiously, the popularity that their concepts enjoyed was not reflected in any increased attention to the category. Although Abraham had a great interest in differentiation, certainly present in his pre-analytic work on the development of the chick, Klein did little to elaborate on category distinctions. On the contrary, mechanisms supposedly specific to manic-depression were described across the diagnostic board. The great irony of Klein's work is that it is essentially a brilliant theory of manic-depression applied to all other clinical structures, yet the international success of the theory did not produce any renewed scrutiny of nosology.

The early American analysts were more focused here, exploring the clinical category and trying to formulate it using Freudian concepts. Ultimately, they were to knock up against the same problems that had bedevilled the psychiatrists. The research group on manic-depression run by Frieda Fromm-Reichmann from 1944 to 1947 at the Washington School of Psychiatry would conclude that "Our investigation led us to question the justification of Kraepelin's classification of the manic-depressive disorder as a specific clinical entity of its own" (Cohen, Baker, Cohen, Fromm-Reichmann, & Weigert, 1954, pp. 103–137). Indeed, the same reclassification seen in psychiatric studies would occur in the analytic ones.

If Jones could cite a 1907 case treated by Otto Gross as the first example of analytic work with a manic-depressive patient, he would later point out that it was, in fact, a case of dementia praecox. Even Jones' case was not immune. Jung immediately sensed that it was also a dementia praecox, and five years later the psychiatrist John MacCurdy asked the hospital to consult its records, confirming Jung's opinion (MacCurdy, 1925, p. 306).

A similar fate awaited the longest and most detailed study of manic-depression to be published within the ambit of Freud's circle, the monograph on 'Flight of Ideas' that Ludwig Binswanger brought out in 1932. Several hundred pages of the minute analysis of the speech of a manic patient are followed by a discreet appendix in which we learn that later events showed that he was in fact schizophrenic, with ideas of influence and hallucinations (Binswanger 1932/2000).

By 1951, Bertram Lewin could state in 'The Psychoanalysis of Elation' that "many deny that there is a manic-depressive psychosis" and that "What seems to be well-understood now is that the old emphasis on the up-and-down swings of mood was obscuring more important psychological issues" (Lewin, 1951, p. 45). What could these issues be?

*

Let's start with mania. In his seminar on 'Dread', discussing the relations between *a* and *i(a)*, Lacan points out that "in mania, it is the non-function of *a*, and no longer simply its misrecognition, which is at stake. It's that something in which the subject is no longer ballasted by any *a*, which delivers him, sometimes without any possibility of freedom, to the pure, infinite and ludic metonymy of the signifying chain" (July 3, 1963).

Now, this comment seems to raise more problems than it solves. How would this non-function of *a* differ from the so-called 'word salad' that we sometimes find in schizophrenia or any of the other language phenomena in psychoses where the signifying chain lacks the support of an object? Secondly, the idea that in mania the signifying chain is infinite and ludic seems clinically incorrect. The most obvious feature of the manias is that, precisely, they stop. As Patty Duke observed when asked what is worse for kids, manias, or depression: "neither, of course, is easy but at least with the manias, my children knew there would be an end within a reasonable period of time. They knew that the mania would stop" (Duke & Hochman, 1992, p. 208).

Likewise, as many analytic and psychiatric students of mania have shown, it is highly structured. What seems to be an infinite and ludic play is in fact, when listened to carefully, restricted in its concerns and follows an underlying logic (see Binswanger, 1932/2000 & Liepmann, 1904). Clang associations, for example, are actually quite rare. The chain is neither infinite nor inherently ludic, although the penchant for humour, punning and verbal jest may sometimes be pronounced, and requires explanation.

As for the non-function of *a*, one would then have to explain how it is that manias end and so-called free intervals can occur: does *a* start to function once again? Can *a* be integrated into *i(a)* as it can in mourning? If *a* is a result of a structural construction of subjectivity, how could it function and then not function? There is the risk here of falling into the trap of seeing mania as what happens to language if you remove the *a*, as if this simply made the subject the puppet of purely associative links between words, exactly the misconception that students of mania like Falret, Liepmann and Binswanger had done their best to dispel. We would be moving towards rather than away from Greisinger's famous definition of mania as a state in which "the soul is free, no longer bound by anything".

But let's stay with the idea of non-function. Doesn't it illuminate certain clinical phenomena here? It is striking how often we hear from manic-depressive subjects about their efforts at housecleaning, and there can be hardly any memoir of manic-depression that does not include some mention of this activity. Something has to be extracted, and if the function of *a* consists, in a sense, in its removal, such activities, which extend from excising dirt to excising part of the brain via ECT, show a certain coherence.

In his memoir of manic-depression, Andy Behrman (2002) describes the strange gratification he would feel when vacuuming up dust balls and detritus in his home, and sweeping the dirt into a neat pile, "an act with a purpose and an end result" (pp. 217–218). This operation of segregation and then extraction mirrors quite precisely his experience of ECT: "Like the hard concrete that filled my brain has been liquefied and drained from my skull" (p. 226).

The tempering effects of the removal of dirt and 'hard concrete' contrast with the extreme vitalisation of the body and the senses in manic-depression. For Terri Cheney (2008), "The slightest sensation feels like a volcanic eruption", it "lights up every nerve ending" (p. 212). While for Behrman (2002), "Sounds are crystal clear, and life appears in front of you on an oversized movie screen", "my eyelashes fluttering on the pillow sound like thunder" (p. xxi). One could read such descriptions of sensory intensification as indications of the non-function of *a*: with its extraction, life will seem less vibrant, less alive. The problem here, once again, is differential: why is it that where the manic-depressive can celebrate this porosity of sensory boundaries (at least at the start of mania), for the schizophrenic it can be a source of absolute terror: sounds are too loud, touch goes too deep, tastes are too strong.

Lacan's point about non-function, if we take a different perspective here, is simply to make mania appear as the opposite of the process by which *a* does function as the support of the signifying chain: called in Seminar 10 desire. Mania and desire represent polarities, depending on the place of the object. Strictly speaking, the reference is to mania rather than to manic-depression. The comments in 'Television' nuance the earlier idea, and form part of a series of references in 1973 in the introduction to the German translation of 'Ecrits' and 'L'Etourdit' (Lacan, 2001, pp. 487, 526, 556).

Speaking of affect in 'Television', Lacan remarks that sadness, which people 'qualify' as depression, is "simply a moral failing, as Dante, and indeed Spinoza, put it: a sin, which means a moral weakness, which is ultimately located only in relation to thought, that is the duty of speaking well (*bien dire*), to situate oneself in relation to the unconscious, to structure. And if ever this weakness, as rejection of the unconscious, ends in psychosis, there's the return in the Real of what is rejected, that is, language: it's the manic excitation by which such a return becomes fatal" (Lacan, 2001, p. 526).

The surprising description of depression as a moral weakness would have raised no eyebrows within the context of Christian ethics. Medieval debates on accidie focused first on whether it was a sin, and, if so, what kind, and later on accidie as negligence of a higher good. Gloom becomes sinful only when we recognise that we are called to God and that hope and joy are duties linked to attainment. Sadness becomes a sin when opposed to the duty of rejoicing in God, and can hence be classed along with hatred, envy, pride and anger.

The duty here is not the Christian life, however, but that of '*bien dire*' and 'finding oneself' in the unconscious, and the most extreme forms of rejection of this are equated with psychosis, a categorical not wanting to know about the unconscious. The fact that it is Dante here rather than St Thomas whom Lacan evokes, is perhaps due to the former's famous opposition in the fifth circle between accidie and the ability to speak: hymns gurgle in the throats of these wretches, for they "cannot speak it in full words".

The reference to mania here is curious. The rejection of locating oneself in relation to the unconscious may offer a definition of psychosis, but why mania? As Colette Soler (2002) points out, Lacan does not say mania here but 'manic excitation' which could be taken in a much more general sense, as indicating any return of libido in the body (pp. 81–96). But again, this is non-specific: why would it take the form of manic excitation rather than any of the myriad forms of morbid agitation and intrusion found, for example, in schizophrenia? Or indeed, following the formula that what is rejected from the symbolic returns in the Real, why not in the form of hallucination?

As to its 'fatal' aspect, it is well known that manic excitation rarely leads to death. On the contrary, suicide is more likely in the depressive phases, and more likely still in times of apparent convalescence. Whatever we make of these details, Lacan's comment still leaves little ambiguity as to his position in the analytic debate on mania: here it is clearly an effect of foreclosure rather than, as Abraham, Rado, Klein and many others believed, a defence against its effects.

But why mania in some cases and not others? We should return here to the work of the early alienists, and separate states of excitation, elation and agitated confusion from mania as such. Loquacity, grandiosity, and the apparent absence of 'guiding ideas' are hardly hallmarks of mania. Real mania does, however, have certain parameters, that I have explored elsewhere: the initial sense that 'The right words are there', that one has a position from which to speak, the necessity of an addressee, the intense feeling of a connection to the world, the conviction that supplies won't run out, the oscillation of a fault, and the rigid separation of binaries, most frequently 'good' and 'bad' (Leader, 2013).

As the arc of mania continues, speech becomes more difficult. Barriers, obstacles and frustrations become magnified. The world "seems to be on a different page". And this brings us to the vital question of how manic episodes end. Lacan (1932/1973) had an interest in this problem in his early psychiatric work and suggested that ideas of persecution played a role here. Clinically this is borne out by the fact that the periods that follow mania so often contain repetitive thoughts of someone 'bad', and it is difficult not to guess that these have a stabilising rather than an aggravating function.

*

If we turn now to the differentiation of the psychoses, we find perhaps more questions than answers. Paranoia, melancholia and the group of the schizophrenias can be separated using the variables of meaning, localisation of libido and distance from the Other. For the paranoiac, the world has a sense: he has succeeded – via delusion – in giving meaning to the desire of the Other. Libido has been localised in the Other, making the paranoiac subject innocent and the Other guilty. Distance to the Other has been regulated, as there is a clear separation between self and Other.

In schizophrenias, in contrast, meaning has not been fixed. Despite the efforts at delusional construction, the question of meaning remains open, and the subject is often suspended there. Libido is not localised in the Other but returns in the subject's mind and body. Boundaries between self and Other may be indistinct and unreliable, and the schizophrenic is often engaged in the lifelong task of trying to maintain them in any way possible.

As for melancholia, the problem of meaning is generally fixed: the subject is guilty. Libido submerges the ego, as we see in the pervasive self-reproach and devaluation, and the relation of self to Other takes the form of the equation that Freud discovered in 'Mourning and Melancholia'. When we turn to manic-depression, things become trickier. As Henri Ey (1954) pointed out, the subject's productions do not seem as anchored in beliefs as, say, those of the paranoiac (p. 55). This, indeed, led some commentators to deny the presence of delusion in manic-depression altogether, or to separate 'manias with delusion' from manias 'without'.

If anything is consistent at the level of sense here, it is less that the Other contains something bad than that the Other is in danger. The altruism of manic episodes and the well-known devotion to charitable and environmental projects are forms of saving the Other, of keeping the Other from harm. Where for the paranoiac the Other harbours a point of toxicity and must be denounced, for the manic-depressive it must, on the contrary, be restored, like the damaged church for St Francis.

Klein recognised this preoccupation in manic-depression yet linked it too hastily to the subject's own aggressive tendencies: the Other was being protected ultimately from oneself. Yet case after case suggests that what is at stake here is not merely the subject's death wishes but the question of a responsibility for death, situated earlier in the family history. A death or tragedy in a previous generation has never been properly inscribed, and so the weight of responsibility hits the subject in the lows and evaporates in the highs. The Other must be kept from danger or declared 'Not Guilty'. Where the paranoiac and melancholic have resolved this question – 'The Other is guilty' and 'I am guilty' respectively – in manic-depression the fault oscillates from the subject to the Other and back again.

Doesn't this also help us to explain the curious vacillations around the sense of identity in manic-depression? One of the most frequently voiced questions is whether it is some kind of foreign body or an intrinsic part of the self. "How much of me is me", asks Lizzie Simon (2002), "and how much of me is the illness?" (p. 210) Would the person really be themselves after the proposed chemical excision of their mania? Do the highs and lows reveal or obscure who they really are? Should manic-depression be seen as constituting or as compromising the self?

The remarkable ubiquity of these questions perhaps echoes the underlying uncertainty about responsibility. Not knowing whether the manias and depressions belong to them or not reflects the difficulty of not knowing whether the responsibility is theirs or someone else's. The hyperidentification with the Other means that the fault is both theirs and the Other's, but never entirely their own. Note the way that, as Duke puts it, in mania "I never really accomplished anything that I could call my own" (Duke & Hochman, 1992, p. 158). And isn't the most common thought after a manic episode precisely to ask, 'What have I done?' Any analytic approach has to explore the reference of this 'I', charting its movement from subject to Other and back again.

Although suicide in manic-depression can occur for a number of different reasons, it can sometimes aim to settle this agonisingly open question of responsibility. Law codes frequently treat suicide as a crime here, yet it would be more accurate to see it, as early English and Roman law did, less as a crime than as a means to eradicate a crime. When the manic-depressive subject appeals for pharmacological or surgical help, it is often to "wipe the slate clean", as if a single act could absolve them, rather like Behrman's vacuuming away of dust and dirt.

If we turn now to the question of libido, it returns for the manic-depressive, as for the schizophrenic, in the body, but also surely in language, although one could make the same claim for many cases of schizophrenia in which the chain of words is a source of libido, either as an enjoyment or as a mortifying, intrusive vehicle. Cheney (2008) makes the brilliant point here that the bodily excitation she experienced was no more and no less than an effect of language: the constant jiggling, movement and physical tension of mania were for her simply forms of the pressure to speak, experienced directly in the body (p. 68).

As for the distance from the Other, this takes on a benign rather than a malignant quality: the subject is joined to the world in a beatific harmony, or at least at the start of the manic arc. There is an acute sense of participation in the Other, understood by many post-Freudians as a stakeholding in the imagined omnipotence of the love object. The fact that it is the Other rather than the other is reflected in the choice of impersonal bodies such as Nature or Civilisation or The Universe, which the subject feels deeply a part of, rather like Sister Maria at the beginning of 'The Sound of Music'.

These are not the only features that may encourage the separation of manic-depression from other forms of psychosis. The phenomena of thought insertion, thought withdrawal and feelings of influence seem to be absent, suggesting that the topological relation with the Other is in marked contrast with schizophrenia. And yet, at the same time, we find plenty of cases where these phenomena are inverted: the person believes during the mania that they are influencing others and transmitting their thoughts to them, just as the sense of identity can undergo strange mutations.

For students of mania like Greisinger and Ey, there was always an 'as if' quality here. The manic-depressive subject somehow never quite believed in the role they were playing out, yet this view may be the result of other factors. The lability of beliefs, which indicated to them the absence of delusional fixity, may simply be a consequence of the need to keep the Other present, alive and out of danger.

For Fromm-Reichman, a schizophrenic subject may be less afraid of attacking this Other because they are less afraid of loneliness. In her terms, the manic-depressive, unlike the schizophrenic, has not accepted the bad mother as his fate (Cohen et al., 1954, p. 126). He can sell out his ideals to gain love. Note the way that hospitalised manic-depressive subjects so frequently manage to gain small privileges on the ward, thereby making themselves special for the nurse or warden they interact with. Where analysts once saw as a sign of orality the fact that admission of manic-depressive subjects would inevitably be followed by a request for a meal, we can understand it here as another example of a small favour to be granted.

The subject here may dispense with surface ideals that have apparently oriented their projects, but the weight of the Other's ideal will always be present. This could take the form of a parental expectation about the child's future, and the subject tries often desperately not to disappoint it. The absolute character of the ideal here has often been noticed by analysts. From a Kleinian perspective, since the subject has to keep good and bad apart, objects can become terrifyingly moral and exacting. Where others located here an accentuation of superego function, the pressure to be perfect which proves so ravaging for the manic-depressive subject can be seen as simply a consequence of this separation of predicates.

There are plenty of cases, likewise, in which mania elevates the subject to a divine position, but, in contrast to other examples, it is always within a nexus of participation: a god to know other gods, or to recognise the godlike in their fellow human beings. The fact that these ideas can so easily be contested after the manic arc has run its course or been arrested chemically perhaps confirms the logical priority of the subject's relation to the Other, so often idealised, rather than to their own insignificance.

It is crucial for the manic-depressive subject to guarantee the Other's belief in them, and this sheds light on the remarkable frequency of Truman Show ideas, in which the person is part of an experiment. Whereas for others the idea that the world is staged for them usually has a menacing quality – to trick them, deceive them, etc. – in manic-depression it is once again benign: it is part of a test to help them move to another level, it is something they are in on. The Other includes them, believes in them and wants them to go forward.

We see this illustrated in the idea, voiced by a manic-depressive patient, that the reality around her was a vast illusion, created to test her: it had all been made up, she said, and she would eventually arrive at the thought that she herself had been made up. Rather than dismissing this as simply a bizarre quirk of psychosis, why not read it as the logical consequence of the structure of manic-depression itself: that the Other's belief has to be maintained at all costs, even at the price of according oneself an illusory status.

Mania here can hardly be identified as a direct effect of foreclosure, even if manic excitation can be. Its function must be restorative, a 'flight into object relations' as it was once called. The idealisations at play can be quite remarkable, and as Fromm-Reichman observed, whereas for many schizophrenic subjects the Other has feet of clay, for the manic-depressive there will be a continued elevation of at least one person to a position of authority or wisdom.

To conclude, I've done my best to sketch out some possible differences between manic-depressive psychosis and the other forms we are familiar with. It seems important to distinguish real mania from the many varieties of excitement and elation that can be mistaken for it. Once we recognise its particularity, the real question is whether we should annex it to the schizophrenias or accord it a separate status.

For my tuppence worth, I would be tempted to include it, primarily because of the forms of mediation employed in relation to the Other. We see so many of the classic features of schizophrenia in reverse that, it is difficult not to infer that the same space of overproximity is in question. The different forms of schizophrenia can then be understood as different ways to manage this space. The ideas of persecution at the beginning and end of manic episodes that Lacan drew attention to in 1932 can be recognised as attempts to reinforce the boundary between self and Other, a boundary that is continually in jeopardy in such a space.

References

Baillarger, J. (1854). Note sur un genre de folie dont les accès sont caractérisés par deux périodes régulières, l'une de dépression, l'autre d'excitation. *Bulletin de l'Académie impériale de médecine, 19*, 382–400.

Behrman, A. (2002). *Electroboy: A Memoir of Mania*. New York: Random House.

Binswanger, L. (2000). *Sur la fuite des idées*. Paris: Millon. (Original work published 1932).

Bleuler, E. (1922). Die probleme der schizoidie und der syntonie. *Zeitschrift für die gesamte Neurologie und Psychiatrie, 78*, 373–399.

Cheney, T. (2008). *Manic: A Memoir*. New York: Harper.

Cohen, M. B., Baker, G., Cohen, R. A., Fromm-Reichmann, F., & Weigert, E. (1954). An intensive study of twelve cases of manic-depressive psychosis. *Psychiatry, 17*, 103–137.

Courbon, P. (1913). Demence precoce et psychose maniaco-depressive: contribution a l'etude des psychoses associees. *Encephale*, May, 434–436.

Duke, P., & Hochman, G. (1992). *A Brilliant Madness: Living with Manic-depressive Illness*. New York: Bantam.

Ey, H. (1954). *Etudes Psychiatriques*, Vol. 3. Paris: Decslée de Brouwer.

Falret, J.-P. (1854). Mémoire sur la folie circulaire. *Bulletin de l'Académie impériale de médecine, 19*, 382–400.

Freud, S. & Jones, E. (1993). *The Complete Correspondence of Sigmund Freud and Ernest Jones*. A Paskauskas (Ed.). Cambridge, MA: Harvard University Press, 263.

Gaupp, R. (1925), Die Frage der kombinierten Psychosen. *Archiv fur Psychiatrie und Nervenkrankheiten, 76*, 73–80.

Hoch, P., & Rachlin, H. L. (1941). An evaluation of manic-depressive psychosis in the light of follow-up studies. *American Journal of Psychiatry, 97*, 831–843.

Jones, E. (1911). Psychoanalytic notes on a case of hypomania. *American Journal of Insanity, 2*, 203–218.

Kraepelin, E. (1920). The manifestations of insanity. *History of Psychiatry, 3*, 1992, 509–529.

Lacan, J. (1973). *De la psychose paranoiaque dans ses rapports avec la personnalite*. Paris: Seuil. (Original work published 1932).

Lacan, J. (2001). *Autres Ecrits*. Paris: Seuil.

Leader, D. (2013). *Strictly Bipolar*. London: Hamish Hamilton.

Lewin, B. (1951). *The Psychoanalysis of Elation*. London: Hogarth.

Liepmann, H. (1904). *Über Ideenflucht*. Halle: Marhold.

MacCurdy, J. (1925). *The Psychology of Emotion*. London: Kegan Paul.

Simon, L. (2002). *Detour: My Bipolar Road Trip in 4-D*. New York: Simon & Schuster.

Soler, C. (2002). La Manie: Peche Mortel. In *L'Inconscient a Ciel Ouvert de la Psychose* (pp. 81–96). Toulouse: Presses Universitaires du Mirail.

Chapter 12

Depression screening as the latest avatar of moralism in American public mental health

Thomas Svolos

When we think of the world as "globalized"—implying a kind of uniform standardization of practices, especially in something such as the psy field, the mental health field—it can be a shock to realize the significant differences between two such equally "advanced Western capitalist" countries such as France and the United States on a matter such as depression screening. Depression screening is currently under debate in France, as a number of forces are pushing France to adopt this practice.

The shock is that depression screening in the United States is something of a *fait accompli*, an established part of the practice of so many clinicians and clinics, schools and universities, and workplaces and community agencies. There is no debate in the United States on this topic, it has been decided—it is a good practice for the mental health field.

Depression screening in the United States can be traced back to 1991, the first National Depression Screening Day (NDSD). This day was established by Screening for Mental Health, Inc., with the financial backing of major pharmaceutical corporations. The non-profit corporation responsible for guiding the NDSD is currently led by a Board of Directors, largely comprising academic psychiatrists. This practice of depression screening was initially promoted to clinicians, but screening—either in person or by the completion of questionnaires, and now online—has been extended to mental health clinicians and clinics, primary care clinics, schools, and workplaces. It is taught in psychiatry residencies and promoted by the US Preventative Services Taskforce recommendations as a "best practice" in medical practice.

Interestingly, while many academics and administrators wish to resolve debates in mental health practice on the grounds of evidence—this whole movement for Evidence-Based Medicine attempts to apply a very reduced Anglo-American "empiricism" in the care of patients to the exclusion of any other values or ethics—there is little significant evidence to support this practice of depression screening. One of the major resources in the analysis of scientific evidence is the Cochrane Library, which provides an online database reviewing the medical literature. In a comprehensive meta-analysis of all the published studies on depression screening to date, they concluded that there is little evidence in support of

DOI: 10.4324/9781003216391-13

this practice. The Summary is unambiguous: "The use of depression screening or case finding instruments has little or no impact on the recognition, management or outcome of depression in primary care or the general hospital" (Gilbody, House, and Sheldon, 2005).

That said, the practice remains in place and well established. There is little debate on this within the psychiatric literature. In the popular literature, such as on the internet, the only critical discussion of this topic can be found in the Scientology literature—with its strong anti-psychiatric positions—and in some comments suggesting that this whole endeavor is supported and funded by the pharmaceutical industry as a way of promoting the diagnosis of depression and subsequent prescription of antidepressants.

Certainly, this latter relationship is important. The Medical-Industrial Complex (of corporations and the physicians who work for them, consult for them, and receive funding from them for their research) has come under increasing scrutiny in the United States at the beginning of the 21st century for hiding negative effects of medications; suppressing unfavorable studies and data that failed to support its products; promoting "off-label" uses of medications for treatments without established benefit; providing excessive payments to physicians by corporations in money and gifts; and, creating a loss of critical scrutiny of the scientific literature due to the overly close relations of researchers to the corporations. We might certainly look upon the pharmaceutical connection to depression screening as just another effort to market their drugs to the public under the rubric of a public health effort, something which would have been necessary for the 1990s, as it was only recently that corporations were allowed to market their drugs directly to the general population through the media.

But there is yet another dimension of this that we must consider, namely the support of employers—including and especially some very large corporations—for this screening. The 1990 Global Burden of Disease Project identified depression as the number one cause of disability in the world and suggested that psychiatric diagnoses were significantly underestimated as a cause of disability. This study has led to additional research in psychiatry in what we might refer to as psycho-economics, namely the effect on the productivity of psychiatric diagnoses such as depression. Large corporations have taken significant notice of this and have implemented depression screening in their workplaces to promote better productivity, enhance workplace safety, and reduce medical and disability expenses.

While the goals of better health and fewer accidents are certainly laudable, we cannot fail to notice another dimension to these practices, which I would identify as an extension of Taylorism into the psyche or mind. In the first industrial era, workers were hired and worked perhaps several different positions within a factory, passing on their knowledge of production to each other. The innovations of Frederick Taylor were to improve efficiency within the factory through scientific management, especially in the analysis of the activities of the workers within the factory, who would subsequently be trained precisely what to do, which often led to the increased specialization of tasks within the factory and greater control by the corporation of their activity. Depression screening, as part of the wellness movement in general so prevalent today in the United States, is nothing other than an extension of the Taylorist doctrine into the minds of the workers themselves—their mental activity is monitored, analyzed, and studied; and, workers are instructed as to the proper state of mind for their jobs. What Fredric Jameson in *Postmodernism, or the Cultural Logic of Late Capitalism* described as one of the last of the pre-capitalist enclaves (the unconscious, along with nature) is now directly territorialized by corporations.

There is yet another dimension, however, to depression screening. One of the sponsoring groups for depression screening is Mental Health America. This non-profit group is an extensive network of organizations with the mission "of promoting mental health, preventing mental disorders, and achieving victory over mental illness through advocacy, education, research, and service." The organization sponsors mental health awareness programs, is a major promoter of screenings, and advocates for care for people with mental illness. The group is one of the largest non-profit groups in the mental health field, and one of the oldest, having been founded originally as the National Committee for Mental Hygiene in 1909 by Clifford Beers, whose story is strikingly close to that of Daniel Paul Schreber. Beers was a very intelligent and educated man, hospitalized in 1900 for a number of years for paranoia. He was subsequently released and wrote an autobiographical account of his life and the poor treatment by the staff in the hospitals where he was confined, *A Mind That Found Itself.* This text led to significant reform in mental health practices and the promotion of a notion of mental hygiene (See Edward Shorter's *A History of Psychiatry* for a brief discussion with references [Shorter, 1997]).

This mental hygiene movement, of which depression screening is the latest manifestation, can be squarely situated within that movement at the turn of the twentieth-century and is described as the Progressive Era (Hofstadter's The Age of Reform [1954] remains a key reference). One aspect of the Progressive agenda that we find in Beers' work and the mental hygiene movement is the notion of social justice and equality for all, with a special focus and reliance on organization and bureaucracy, with the support of science, to achieve these changes. The Progressive Era is often described as a response to the rapid changes occurring at that time in history and is mostly associated with industrialization. For example, Upton Sinclair's 1906 *The Jungle*, which chronicled the abuses of the workers in the meat packing industry, led to bureaucratic initiatives such as the Food and Drug Administration, which regulated food through a systematization of food production as an industry. Beers' books similarly took issue with the increasingly "factory-like" nature of the American asylums of the time, where he was confined. The crucial logic for all of these efforts, however, was a notion of what we might even term an Aristotelian Sovereign Good, be it in the care of animals or patients in asylums, that holds true for society—for everyone in society—and one which must be secured through the action of government, enlisting the help of science, in promotion of this Good for all.

There is yet a further historical antecedent for this in the first half of the nineteenth century in the United States—the period known as the Second Great Awakening. The history of the United States has been marked by various periods of heightened religious activity, periods of great interest in protestant evangelism, and times that are often referred to as Great Awakenings. The second one, though, from 1800–1835, is most notable, as in addition to the personal religious dimension present in the earlier Great Awakening, this latter movement is notable for various reform causes – efforts to bring rights and equality to women and blacks (through the women's suffrage movement and the abolition movement) and, important in the context of depression screening, the development of the temperance movement and movements against masturbation and sexuality as such, which brought religion into personal behavior in a public and universal way for all (and eventually resulted, in the later Progressive Era, in the Constitutional Amendment of Prohibition, which banned the production and sale of alcohol for a number of years).

A review article by Jill Lepore on the Second Great Awakening discussed the historical debate on the relationship of these reform efforts to the growth of egalitarian Jacksonian democracy and the expansion of American business (Lepore, 2007). Cited in Lepore, Charles Sellers' *The Market Revolution: Jacksonian America, 1815–1846* argues for the importance of this period as the critical moment of a shift from an agrarian to a market capitalist economy, during which "Establishing capitalist hegemony over economy, politics, and culture, the market revolution created ourselves and most of the world we know." Sellers' thesis is strongly disputed by Daniel Walker Howe's *What Hath God Wrought: The Transformation of America, 1815–1848*, but both acknowledge a historical transition during this period. As Lepore succinctly summarizes it: "Sellers thinks that poor, drunk, lusty, impious eighteenth-century Americans were freer, and happier, than their wealthier, sober, prim, devout nineteenth-century grandchildren; Howe thinks it's the grandchildren who were better off."

What strikes one immediately with a chronology such as this, however, from the Second Great Awakening to the Progressive Era to the depression screening of today, is how each of these moral reform efforts—within the mental health field: from temperance and movements against sexuality to mental hygiene to depression screening—occurs at a pivotal moment in American economic history: the transition to a market economy, the transition to monopoly capitalism and, now, the development of advanced or global capitalism. Each moment carries within it one more effort for a greater morality for all, in a well-nigh Weberian logic, extending moral control from that of behaviors such as drunkenness into the psyche itself, with an increasing alliance with science to bolster these programs, even when science itself offers no support for practices such as depression screening.

This is moralism, writ large on the political stage, and is indeed something that Jacques Lacan warned about, in 1960, in *The Ethics of Psychoanalysis*, stating that:

There is absolutely no reason why we should make ourselves the guarantors of the bourgeois dream. A little more rigor and firmness are required in our confrontation with the human condition. That is why I reminded you last time that the service of goods or the shift of the demand for happiness onto the political stage has its consequences. The movement that the world we live in is caught up in, of wanting to establish the universal spread of the service of goods as far as conceivably possible, implies an amputation, sacrifices, indeed a kind of puritanism in the relationship to desire that has occurred historically. The establishment of the service of goods at a universal level does not in itself resolve the problem of the present relationship of each individual man to his desire in the short period of time between his birth and his death. The happiness of future generations is not at issue here.

(Lacan, 1992, p. 303)

Lacan may well have been describing moralism in mental health in its American manifestations. It is a valuable cautionary note for all clinicians today, whether psychoanalysts or not.

References

Gilbody, S., House, A. O., & Sheldon, T. A. (2005) Screening and case finding instruments for depression. *Cochrane Database of Systematic Reviews*, 4, 19 October.

Lacan, J. (1992). *The Seminar of Jacques Lacan: Book VII, The Ethics of Psychoanalysis 1959–1960*. New York: Norton.

Lepore, J. (2007) Vast designs: How America came of age. *The New Yorker*, 29 October.

Shorter, E. (1997). *A History of Psychiatry: From the Era of the Asylum to the Age of Prozac*. New York: John Wiley and Sons.

Index

For Product Safety Concerns and Information please contact our EU
representative GPSR@taylorandfrancis.com
Taylor & Francis Verlag GmbH, Kaufingerstraße 24, 80331 München, Germany

www.ingramcontent.com/pod-product-compliance
Lightning Source LLC
Chambersburg PA
CBHW050650280326
41932CB00015B/2850

* 9 7 8 1 0 3 2 1 0 6 5 3 3 *